QUIT
SKINNY!

7 SIMPLE, SANE
STEPS TO WELLNESS

QUIT SKINNY!

7 SIMPLE, SANE STEPS TO WELLNESS

CONNIE R. CLAY

SHE FLOURISHES, INC. · JACKSONVILLE, FL.

QUIT SKINNY! 7 SIMPLE, SANE STEPS TO WELLNESS

Requests for information should be addressed to:
She Flourishes, Inc.
P.O. Box 77220
Jacksonville, FL 32226

All Internet addresses were current and accurate at the time of publication; however, the addresses and content of these resources may change. The mentioning of these Internet addresses is not intended as an endorsement, and the author and publisher do not vouch for the content of these sites for the life of this book.

Quit Skinny! contains the ideas and opinions of the author. This book is not a substitute for medical advice or treatment. This book is for the purpose of education and information, and it is not a substitute for treatment from a medical professional. You should consult a physician before you begin this or any wellness or exercise program. Neither the author nor the publisher shall be liable for any damage that allegedly arises from the use of any information in this book.

Additional copies of this book are available at www.ConnieClay.com.

Publisher's Cataloging-in-Publication data

Clay, Connie Renee.
    Quit skinny ! 7 simple , sane steps to wellness / Connie R. Clay.
    p. cm.
    ISBN 978-0-9903892-0-0
    Includes bibliographical references and index.

    1. Women—Health and hygiene. 2. Self-care, Health. 3. Physical fitness. 4. Mind and body. 5. Weight loss—Psychological aspects. 6. Overweight women—Psychology. 7. Body image. I. Quit skinny ! seven simple , sane steps to wellness. II. Title.
    RA776.95.C6 2014
    613—dc23   2014908559

Cover design by: ArrowDesign; arrowdesigns01@gmail.com
Interior design by: Elizabeth A. Blacker, elizabethblacker@me.com

DEDICATION

I dedicate this book to my parents, Carnell Clay and the late Rayphield Clay. God used you to bring me into this world. Thank you for loving me, nurturing me, scolding me and demanding that I make something of myself.

CONTENTS

INTRODUCTION

"The first wealth is health."

—Ralph Waldo Emerson

Millions of women struggle to be physically well. We suffer from diabetes, heart disease, cancer, and other illnesses that are linked to our lifestyle. As women, we're busy. We work, take care of the children and elders, and try to manage the household. So how do we find the time to take care of our bodies? We don't. We put ourselves in last place. Several years ago, I was diagnosed with prediabetes. I've tried dozens of weight-loss programs in my lifetime. Many of these programs promised that I would lose weight quickly and keep it off. But these quick-fix plans left me fatter, broker, and sicker.

I spent over 20 years putting my family and career ahead of my health. I ended up unhappy and unhealthy. This book started with notes to myself on my phone, about what was helping me to become well and what was not working. After several months, I realized that others could benefit from my findings.

I know. You've tried every program in the world to lose weight. You've even tried plans that claimed you could eat whatever you want, not exercise, and still lose weight. But these programs left you with less money, more weight, and more frustration. If you've peeked at the basics of this plan and you're still reading, that's great news for both of us!

So why does this plan work? For starters, it's simple. I didn't say it was easy, but it is a simple program. This wellness program is not a quick fix. It is a series of gradual changes that will last forever. Many of my suggestions are backed by scientific research. I have tried everything I am suggesting to you and much more. This book is the best of my 30 plus years of trial and error. Most of the food that you will eat is the best food on the planet for mental and physical wellness. No food is off limits. I think when we say that certain foods are never ever allowed, those foods become that much more attractive.

Is this another diet?

I know what you're thinking! Oh no, not another diet. This is not a diet! I hate diets, being deprived, and being hungry. This is a program to help you get healthy, well, fit, or however you choose to describe feeling great. I began to see some progress with my fitness goals when I decided that being healthy was my first priority. Yes, you have to work hard. But you don't ever again have to diet.

Diets don't work. I've been on enough of them to know that with 100% certainty. It usually goes like this. You have your "last" supper on Sunday, which means you go to a buffet and eat all the things you won't be able to eat on your diet. Monday comes and you have some sort of protein shake for breakfast. You have a tiny little lunch and convince yourself you've had enough to eat. Your afternoon snack is something you either don't like or are indifferent about, such as cauliflower. Dinner is something that no one else in your house will eat. Dessert is a gelatin or pudding that is artificially sweetened. After three days of this torture, you go and grab a burger and fries for lunch. It's so good to be satisfied! And then you tell yourself you're fat, lazy, and undisciplined. Sound familiar?

This wellness plan is the opposite of a diet. You choose from a variety of healthy foods, drinks, and spices. You take care of your body and your brain. You prepare yummy meals that your family will enjoy and appreciate. Perhaps the best

Don't ever talk down to yourself.

part is that you will feel better. You won't be nervous and cranky. After a few weeks, family and friends will notice something different about you. If you slide back into your old unhealthy habits, there is no shame or guilt. You acknowledge you are human and get back on track.

I don't consider myself a biblical scholar, but I do have a Christ-centered view of life. So I will refer to my Christian faith from time to time because I could not have achieved my wellness goals nor could I have written this book without the love and help of my Lord and Savior, Jesus Christ.

Read the book from cover to cover, or start with the chapter that interests you the most. Love yourself. Give yourself credit for opening the book. Forget what you did or did not do yesterday. You can begin again, and your journey starts now.

I have walked a thousand miles in your shoes. Share your trials and triumphs with me. Email me at Connie@Connie Clay.com. Or connect with me on Facebook.

QUIT SKINNY!

Stop Chasing a Number on the Scale,
and Focus on the Important
Measures of Wellness

*"By choosing healthy over skinny,
you are choosing self-love over
self-judgment. You are beautiful!"*

—STEVE MARABOLI

In December 2009 I reached my highest weight ever, 211 pounds. My BMI (body mass index) was 42.6, which meant that I was morbidly obese. Sounds pretty bad, doesn't it? But how could I be pronounced seriously unhealthy based on two numbers, my height and weight? I had no control of my height, so based on one number over which I had control, I was unhealthy, according to the BMI. The BMI is a grading system that compares height and weight to determine who is underweight, normal, overweight, obese, morbidly obese, or super obese. I had reached that weight despite over 30 years of dieting.

I had also been diagnosed with prediabetes. I had painful arthritis in my hips and knees.

During that time I had trouble sleeping two or three nights a week. So, after all those years of dieting, why was I so unhealthy? Because my focus was wrong. For all those years I longed to weigh 120 pounds, which was completely unrealistic for me. According to the BMI, that's about where I should be, at 4'11" tall. However, I haven't weighed 120 pounds since I was 12 years old!

Stop treating your body like a garbage disposal.

The way I looked and felt was not acceptable. I decided I was going to find or create a system that would allow me to feel better physically and mentally, sidestep my strong family history of diabetes, look better, and lose some weight. I tried a couple more diets and one last quick-weight-loss scheme before I decided to stop aiming for 120 pounds on the scale. I quit skinny.

I am most proud of the fact that once I quit skinny, I lost over 30 pounds. I no longer struggle with insomnia. My endocrinologist (diabetes specialist) released me from his practice and advised me to follow up with my primary care physician. My blood pressure, blood sugar, and lipid levels are perfect.

If you want to check my definition of perfect, research my numbers:
• Blood pressure: 112/57

- Pulse: 62
- Total cholesterol: 158
- HDL (high-density lipoprotein cholesterol, also called "good" cholesterol): 61
- LDL(low-density lipoprotein cholesterol, also called "bad" cholesterol: 78
- Triglycerides (fat carried in the blood): 95
- Blood glucose (about an hour after lunch): 93

These readings were taken at a health fair on August 24, 2013. After reviewing my numbers, the wellness nurse asked me what I did! She pronounced me healthy and told me to keep it up because she had no suggestions for improvement.

Don't aim for perfection; aim for progress.

On this plan, I want you to be well, mentally and physically. You'll have to take the time to retrain yourself. When you're getting enough sleep, exercising on a regular basis, drinking plenty of water, and eating the best foods for health, you will lose some weight and you will greatly increase your chances of living a long and healthy life.

Why Should You Quit Skinny and Focus on Wellness?

I have a few reasons for you. First, the number on the scale is only a number. I have a coworker who is tall and thin and about 30 years old. She has a difficult time with high cholesterol. The coworker has a strong family history of high cholesterol. She is probably at a greater risk of heart

> *Don't settle
> for second rate
> medical care.*

disease than I am. This is only one example of how the scale should not be the sole basis that we use to determine who is healthy and who is not.

A recent article in *Essence* magazine[1] profiled five women. These women varied in size. A couple of them were curvy, one was thin, and one was voluptuous, but based on a "health score," these women were well regardless of whether they were considered skinny or not. The health score was based on their age, height, blood pressure, total cholesterol level, fasting blood sugar, weight, physical activity, tobacco use, and alcohol consumption. For more

> *Wellness is how you
> feel and look and so
> much more than how
> much you weigh!*

information on this process of assessing health and wellness, check out the Johnson & Johnson Digital Health Scorecard which is available in the iTunes Store or Google "Digital Health Scorecard."

A recent study by the National Cancer Institute[2] found that adults who exercised on a regular basis lived longer than those who did not exercise. Even overweight adults who exercised lived longer than their slender counterparts who did not exercise. In an article titled "Can Being Overweight Help You Live Longer?" Melinda Wenner Moyer noted that the BMI is viewed as a

1 "Be Healthy at Every Size," by Gina Roberts-Grey, July 2013.
2 To read the article, go to www.plosmedicine.org. For an overview of the findings, visit http://www.nih.gov/news/health/nov2012/nci-06.htm

flawed standard because it relates weight only to height.[3] Wenner Moyer added that some studies suggest that body fat may have a protective quality if a person is sick. She also reported that those viewed as overweight and obese may receive better health care because doctors may treat obese patients more aggressively. So we see that being thin does not equate to wellness.

How Do We Measure Wellness?

Let's start with how you feel. Really think about it.
- Do you have trouble getting to sleep or staying asleep?
- Are you always tired?
- Are you usually grumpy?
- Are you out of breath after climbing a flight of steps?
- Do your hips, knees, and feet hurt?

Pain lets us know that something is not right. If you are in pain on a regular basis, chances are you are not well. There is no reason to accept pain and discomfort as normal.

For years, I tolerated hip pain and stiffness. My knees were often painful too. I felt that if I discussed these issues with a doctor, I'd get the same old advice, "lose weight." Finally, I made an appointment with an orthopedist. He did a clinical exam and took X-rays. After being diagnosed with degenerative arthritis, I was offered injections for my

3 The article was published in the June 2013 issue of *The Oprah Magazine*.

knees and physical therapy for my hips and knees. I accepted both. I worked with a physical therapist once or twice a week for about six weeks. He taught me exercises that I could do at home and at work, as part of my normal routine. I completed my course of physical therapy several months ago, and I had three injections in each knee about eight months ago. My hips have never felt better. My knees are sometimes sore and swollen, but it's not nearly as bad as it was before I received treatment.

Caution Signs

Is your blood pressure high? Do you have diabetes? Have you been told that you have prediabetes? Do you have problems with acid reflux? These are all indicators that you are not well. So, what is wellness? I define wellness as feeling your best mentally and physically, and being able to engage in activities you enjoy. Some conditions are asymptomatic, so you can't completely rely on how you feel.

> *Get at least 10 minutes of sunshine every day to improve your mental health.*

I tested my wellness on the www.healthcalculators.org website. I also assessed my cardiovascular disease risk by answering a few questions. My risk of having a major cardiovascular event in the next 10 years is 1%. I'll take that!

I recommend seeing a doctor at least twice a year. See your gynecologist once a year for a pelvic exam, Pap smear, and breast exam. Your gynecologist will usually check your blood pressure and pulse. She should ask if you are having any problems or unusual symptoms. Six months after you have the appointment with your gynecologist, have an appointment with your internist. He or she should order fasting blood work to check for diabetes and elevated lipid levels. By staggering these appointments every six months, you could catch some ailments early. See your health care team more often, if recommended. Consider yourself the most important member of your health care team because you are!

Mental Health Matters, Too

Now, if you are always tired, sad, nervous, or grumpy, that's not normal. Definitely review the chapter on sleep. If you're following all the recommendations on this plan and you're still tired, sad, nervous, and/or crabby, you should consult a mental health professional. You may have depression and/or anxiety. If you were walking around with a broken arm, you'd see a doctor, wouldn't you? If your mental health is poor, you should see a professional. You may need some counseling or you may need counseling and medication. Heredity, life events, and environment can cause anyone to experience mental health problems. There is no shame in getting help. There are many resources online and at the library on mental health.[4]

---

4 For a short, easy to understand article about mental health, visit http://www.may oclinic.com/health/mental-health/MH00042/METHOD=print.

So Quit Skinny! Stop believing that being thin means you will be healthy. To be well, you actually have to go deeper than size and weight. You have to assess how you feel physically and mentally. You have to look at blood pressure, blood sugar, and lipid levels. Try one or all of the measures of health mentioned in this chapter to assess where you are and where you would like to be.

QUIT SKINNY NOTES

Use this section to write down ideas, goals, and questions.

_____
_____
_____
_____
_____
_____
_____
_____
_____
_____
_____
_____
_____
_____
_____
_____
_____

Chapter Two

My Dieting Résumé:

Diets and Programs That I Tried and Fired

"Mistakes are a fact of life. It is the response to error that counts."

—Nikki Giovanni

I f I could have a talk with my 12-year-old self, I would tell her that she is delightful, funny, smart, and worthy of love. I would tell her that her being a little chubby is okay. I would tell her to start sleeping well and to find an exercise she enjoys doing. I would tell her to eat lots of fresh fruits and veggies and to plan to study wellness forever. I would urge her to focus on her physical and mental well-being, not how much she weighs. The 12-year-old me was caught in a cycle of self-hate primarily because of her weight.

Stop rushing yourself. It took decades to get unhealthy; allow several months to reverse the damage.

In hindsight, I realize that my grandmother was an island of sanity for me, from my birth until she died, when I was in my late twenties.

My grandmother was my best friend. She accepted me as I was. She never made fun of me or criticized me because of my weight. She was my emotional parent. She loved me unconditionally and she nurtured me. She always made me feel that I could do anything. She also taught me how to bake. For most of the first 12 or 13 years of my life, I spent weekends at my grandmother's home. My great-grandmother, grandmother, great-aunts, and great uncle all lived in our family home in the Oak Grove section of Chesapeake, Virginia. My mother, brother, and I referred to them collectively as "the people in Oak Grove." Every Saturday night, my grandmother baked a pound cake from scratch. As I grew older and had a steady grip, she would allow me to add the sugar, flour, and butter. She would place the cake in a wood-burning stove, and then we would start the homemade yeast rolls. Breakfast on Sunday mornings included fried codfish cakes and those fresh-baked yeast rolls with butter. Just writing about those days brings a smile to my face and comfort to my heart.

Learn how to celebrate without food.

I didn't realize it at the time, but I started associating food with love, comfort, and acceptance. I had always been a little chubby, and I was sensitive about my weight. At the age of 12, I saw an ad for diet pills. I usually had thirty or forty dollars on hand because my grandmother and great-aunts gave me money and I really had no expenses. I bought a money order and ordered the mail-order diet pills. I took the pills to my grandmother's house for the weekend. Thank God she found them and bought them from me. I have no idea what effect those drugs would have had on a 12-year-old in the '70s, when there was less regulation of weight-loss products.

When I was a teenager, my mother signed me up to attend a weight-loss studio in the mall. I went to the weight-loss center after school. I remember lying on a table that vibrated for about 30 minutes. My "customized" diet included oatmeal. I had no success with the program. Decades later, as I look at pictures of myself from high school, I see I wasn't that heavy. I was 4' 11" and my weight was around 135 pounds, but I was convinced I was fat and unacceptable.

I really started gaining weight while in college. I don't remember making an effort to exercise or lose weight during those years. There was so much fun on campus and in the city and so many friends to share life with.

This is a good time to start loving yourself.

I completed college in May 1984, and when I enrolled in law school in August 1984, I was pregnant with my first child, Brittany. I was unmarried, and Brittany's father was uninvolved. My weight was up to about 170 pounds. I had a relatively trouble-free pregnancy and gained only 19 pounds. Afraid of doing something or failing to do something that would harm my unborn child, I kept a log to make sure I ate

> We live in a time where we can easily research what we should and should not put into our bodies.

all my veggies, dairy, meats, and other necessities. I didn't have a car, so I always walked to and from bus stops and anywhere I needed to go that was less than a couple of miles. Brittany weighed in at a respectable eight pounds and one ounce. By the time Brittany was two weeks old, I had lost the 19 pounds gained while pregnant with her. My great-aunt and my mother came to help me after Brittany was born, making it possible for me to resume my studies immediately. I returned to my involuntary walking routine, and I breastfed for a short time, which helped me lose the pregnancy weight effortlessly.

Once I completed law school, I accepted a job at the State Attorney's Office in Jacksonville, Florida, where working 80 hours a week was routine. I was also studying for the bar exam. I had enough time to commute, work, raise my daughter, and repeat the cycle. I knew little about what to eat, what not to eat, or how to maintain a healthy weight.

My mother kept Brittany off and on until I passed the bar. After my first year as a prosecutor, I was promoted to the sex crimes unit. I loved the work, and the hours were much better. I was beginning to have a life away from the office. I remember exercising to a Jane Fonda workout record! Still, even though the bar was behind me and my schedule was more reasonable, I was clueless about health and wellness. My weight was probably up around 190 pounds when I left the State Attorney's Office in 1989.

My next job was in the corporate law offices of an insurance company. My hours were even better than they had been in the sex crimes unit. I started drinking diet shakes and going to a dance aerobics class. I lost about 40 or 50 pounds in a few months and was my slimmest ever as an adult. I was quite pleased with myself. Still, I wanted to lose more. At one point, I was limiting myself to 800 calories a day. During this period of starving myself, I started fainting.

Fortunately, I was always in a safe place when I lost consciousness. At some point, I went to a freestanding weight-loss center. They were advertising a $25.00 special, but the $25.00 only included the vitamins that I "needed." I didn't lose any weight on that program, but I did lose my $25.00. For the next few years, I did a decent job of keeping my weight at around 150 pounds, but I was never satisfied. I wanted to see 120 pounds or less on the scale.

While pregnant with my second daughter in 1995, I gained 28 pounds. I breastfed her for several months and did a decent job of getting back to my pre-pregnancy weight of 150 pounds. This was an acceptable weight. I wish I had maintained it. Instead, I wanted to lose more and ended up gaining more. I wish I had stopped aiming for skinny.

Here are some other things that I tried in order to lose weight.

Scale Minders

For several years, I tried various versions of this established program. What I disliked about all the versions was that the only progress that was rewarded was weight loss. I worked so hard some weeks, only to see that the scale hadn't moved or I had gained weight. I reached my five-pound mark and then had a hard time losing any more weight. I also hated having to write down everything I ate. For me, the worst part about Scale Minders was listening to other participants whine and cry about what they ate that they shouldn't have eaten. Oh, shut up! I thought as I sat there fuming that I had not lost any weight.

Permanent wellness is a slow and gradual process.

I wonder how much money I wasted going to Scale Minders. It occurred to me after the fact that if the program were truly effective, there would be no need for a "lifetime membership." Why would you ever need to go back if the weight loss were permanent? Even though I haven't been to Scale Minders in several years, I receive a postcard a couple of times a year inviting me to come back and rejoin. Why would I do that!

Diet Drugs

In 2011, I decided I would use any means necessary to lose the 50 extra pounds I had carried most of my adult life. A few days before my 49th birthday, I enrolled at a rapid-weight-loss clinic. Although I knew quite a bit about exercise and nutrition by then, I had never consistently applied the principles. My gynecologist owned the weight-loss clinic, so I assumed that all the procedures were safe. I had been a patient at the practice for over 15 years and trusted the doctor and his staff. The nurse-practitioner suggested I try the program. After an EKG, I was pronounced fit enough to get slim with rapid weight loss. A nurse came in to give me two shots. I know one was B12. I trembled as I bent over to get the shots. Something just didn't feel right. The nurse asked me if I was okay. After the shots, she reviewed my diet with me. I was allowed 500 calories a day. A weight-loss drug was prescribed. The nurse assured me that if I took the pills, I would be able to limit myself to 500 calories a day. Next, she gave me a kit to check my urine after a few days to see if ketosis had set in. Ketosis is when the body is so deprived of carbohydrates that it burns fat for energy.

I knew this diet was not medically sound, but I desperately wanted to lose weight. I thought that if I could lose 10–15 pounds on this program, maybe I could do the rest on my own. My insurance company approved the program, and I only had a $30.00 per week co-pay, so it had to be good for me, right? The first couple of days were okay. I was

Don't be afraid to walk away from a bad situation.

adjusting to the tiny caloric intake. I didn't tell anyone I was on the diet because I wanted everyone to be stunned when I started losing weight. One Sunday morning when I had been starving myself and taking the pills for about four days, I felt really light-headed, but I wanted to go to church. I tested my blood sugar, and it was down to 74[5] after I had eaten my tiny breakfast. I had an apple, which wasn't allowed on the plan, but I knew I needed to get my blood sugar up. I still felt light-headed and woozy, but well enough to continue with my day. After church, we went to the mall. I don't remember what I ate. My daughter didn't know what I was doing to myself. I wanted a pretty new dress for my birthday. I didn't find a dress that I liked by the time the mall closed at 6:00 p.m. and was disappointed.

Fear exists only in my head.

When we left the mall, I was tired. I had driven across the Matthews Bridge thousands of times in the 24 years I'd lived in Jacksonville. As we approached the bridge, I got nervous. I told myself I could cross the bridge. Once I got to the top, I panicked. I thought I would lose control of the car. I applied the brakes even though nothing was in front of me. I took deep breaths hoping that I could regain my composure. The panic attack lasted about 30 seconds, but it seemed much longer. Once we were over the bridge, my daughter asked me what was wrong. For the first time, I admitted to myself that I had a panic disorder.

I confided in my daughter that the attacks had been going on for a year. All of the attacks occurred while I was driving. To avoid the panic attacks, I avoided the places where I had panicked. My universe had grown smaller. I could no longer drive over the Hart Bridge, yet I could

---

5 A normal fasting blood sugar reading is between 70–99, and a normal blood sugar reading after meals is between 135–140.

still drive over the Matthews Bridge—until that Sunday. I hadn't told anyone what was happening to me. I was embarrassed and I thought I was too strong to have a mental disorder. After the panic attack, I told my daughter the truth about my diet. She was shocked and disappointed that I had resorted to such drastic measures to lose weight. The panic attack scared her. She didn't know I had kept secrets from her.

The next morning, I called the diet doctor's office to report what had happened. A nurse called back a few hours later. She seemed unconcerned, and offered to call in a different prescription. By that time, I had decided to quit the plan. I met with a physician's assistant at my primary care physician's office and learned that panic attacks are common side effects of diet drugs. Although I had been having panic attacks for a year, I had not experienced one on that bridge. The physician's assistant prescribed Buspar, explaining that it was an antidepressant which could treat anxiety. On my check-out form was the diagnosis: anxiety disorder. I couldn't believe the weight-loss clinic hadn't warned me about the side effects of the drugs. However, I can't say with 100% certainty that I would not have risked the side effects in exchange for rapid weight loss.

Untrained Personal Trainers

I've tried personal training several times. The first time, I enrolled in a group training class at a gym. There were four students and one trainer. The trainer had us begin exercising without warming up. By the third or fourth session, I pulled a quad muscle—quite a painful start. I didn't complete the class. I ended up having to see a doctor and get a prescription muscle relaxer to relieve the pain.

My next attempt at personal training was in the summer of 2010. I found a facility not far from my office. I wanted a female trainer, but a male was available when I called, so I decided to give him a try. I paid $300.00 for a month of personal training sessions. During my first session, the trainer kept looking at his phone and responding to text messages. At the second session, I had a headache. The same thing happened at the third session. My physician found nothing wrong, but told me to stop the training sessions. Based on this advice, I requested a refund for the unused sessions. The owner of the facility refused to refund my money until I threatened to expose her and report her to the Better Business Bureau.

The way it starts out is usually the way it ends up.

About 18 months later, I signed up for a weight-loss program at the gym. For $800.00, I would get one nutrition consultation a week and three personal training sessions a week. I really liked the dietician, Sue, because she seemed to understand the difficulties of trying to establish a healthy eating plan. My personal trainer was Maria. While training me, Maria often looked at her fingernails.

She would demonstrate the exercises once, but wouldn't do them with me, nor would she count the repetitions. Maria told me that she completed nursing school, but in her last semester decided she didn't want to be a nurse. She divulged that she liked being a trainer because she was able to have a free gym membership; yet she dreamed of being a chef. Maria pushed me further than I pushed myself; however, I never achieved the results I wanted while working with her. Maria is now a pastry chef.

Last year, one of my Facebook friends posted that she had lost several dress sizes while working with a personal trainer. I got her trainer's info and signed up. The trainer had recently left the navy. She never disclosed her physical problems, but implied she had some sort of disability. She said she was working on a master's degree. I never inquired about her training or experience. We met at the fitness center in her apartment complex. Although she had me agree to release her from liability if there were any injuries, there was no release for the apartment complex. At the beginning of the second session, while warming up on the treadmill, I started having a headache. Brittany, my oldest daughter, and I have named these events "discernment headaches." By then, I had figured out that this trainer did not have the consent of the apartment complex to conduct personal training in their fitness facility. I knew I couldn't work with her and walk in integrity, so I chose integrity. I haven't had any problems with headaches since then.

Intuitive Eating

Several years ago, a friend told me that she stopped weighing herself, took up ballroom dancing, ate what she wanted, and at the end of three years, had lost 30 pounds. I've heard about programs where you eat what you want, but you stop when you're full. It's called intuitive eating. Maybe that will work for some folks, but it never worked for me. I intuitively wanted 3,000 calories a day, from the wrong foods and drinks, which would not allow me to reach my wellness goals. I wish I could give these programs a thumbs-up, but I never had any success with them.

So there you have it, a summary of all the schemes and programs I tried that did not work.

QUIT SKINNY NOTES

Use this section to write down ideas, goals, and questions.

_____
_____
_____
_____
_____
_____
_____
_____
_____
_____
_____
_____
_____
_____

Chapter Three

7 Simple, Sane Steps to Wellness

"Our life is frittered away by detail. Simplify, simplify."

—Henry David Thoreau

Becoming well is a journey. The Quit Skinny Wellness Plan is based on seven simple steps that anyone can implement.

1. Sleep 7–9 hours a night.

Getting enough rest is as important to your health as what you eat and how much you exercise. I will discuss sleep in more detail in the chapter called "Why Sleep Matters." Your body and mind need rest to function properly. When you deprive yourself of sleep, you will find it difficult to maintain a healthy lifestyle. You may crave carbohydrates and caffeine to get you through the day.

You might be wondering how you'll find time to sleep for seven hours a night. I know it's not easy, but you have to decide that your wellness is a priority. My priorities are as follows: My Christian walk, my physical and mental wellness, my family, and my career. The best gift that I can give my family is a healthy and whole me. Some of the things I do to make room for wellness are to admit that I can't do everything as well as I would like to. Some things have to wait. When deciding how to spend the limited time I have, I consider my priorities.

Let's say I get home at 7:00 p.m. If I didn't spend time with the Lord that morning, I have dinner and then my quiet time with the Lord. By then, it's 8:00 p.m. I go ahead and take 15 minutes to prepare my lunch and prep my breakfast for the next day. If there are bills that need to be paid or other household tasks, I allow 30–45 minutes to do what I can. The world won't end if I don't file all the statements after I pay the bills. I head into the bathroom around 10:00 p.m. to get ready for bed. If I go to bed at 10:30 p.m., I usually set the alarm for 5:30 a.m.

You'll notice that I didn't say anything about playing on Facebook, watching TV, or engaging in other leisurely pursuits. These activities have their place, but on a busy night I choose not to make time for them. My youngest daughter lives at home, so conversations with her occur throughout the evening. We take a few minutes at the end of the night to say family prayer. My oldest daughter will call and claim that she only needs five minutes to talk, but an hour later I'm still on the phone with her!

2. Drink at least 7 glasses of water a day.

If you exhaled loudly, rolled your eyes, or said out loud, "I hate water," I know how you feel. Even though I've made the effort to drink seven glasses a day for the past few years, I still don't enjoy it that much. I'd rather have an ice-cold Coke! However, that Coke does not get me closer to my wellness goals. I have a real Coke twice a year, on my birthday and my half birthday. If you've never heard the term half birthday, it's the date six months before your birthday. I learned this term when my children were younger. I refused to acknowledge and celebrate their half birthdays. But I celebrate mine with a Coke or a frozen Coke.

Our bodies are mostly made of water. We need water for proper brain function, to keep our joints working smoothly, to aid in digestion, and to keep our skin soft and supple.

How do you go from no water to seven glasses a day? Gradually. If you normally drink seven or eight glasses of sweet tea or soda a day, start by diluting one glass with 50% water. This will get you accustomed to drinking less tea or soda and more water. After a few days, you won't mind the water in your tea. At the end of a few days, start having one glass of water. Another way to add water is to make it convenient. Buy a pretty water bottle. Fill it at night and have it ready to go when you leave for work. Sip it on the way to work and sip from it throughout your day. If you exercise, drink a full glass of water before you start, while you're exercising, and have a third glass when you finish. This will replenish the water that you lose while sweating.

3. Eat 3–4 veggies a day and 2–3 fruits a day.

Starchy veggies such as corn and white potatoes are not included because they are high in carbohydrates and not that great in terms of fiber. Eating fresh fruits and veggies will help to prevent constipation and hemorrhoids. Fruits and veggies are excellent sources of fiber, vitamins, nutrients, antioxidants, and water. Once you start adding these nutritional powerhouses to your diet, you will actually crave them. Although fruits do have a decent amount of carbohydrates, the fiber and water in them make them a healthy choice. For suggestions on what fruits and veggies to eat, see the chapter, "What You Should Eat and Drink."

4. Eat 20 Meals a Week from the "What You Should Eat and Drink" chapter.

As you begin your journey to wellness, you will need to make gradual changes in what you eat. Some of my favorite foods are macaroni and cheese, cheesecake, peach pie, and fried catfish. While I love these foods, I limit my intake. I may have a big piece of cheesecake three or four times a year, without any guilt. However, I recognize that I can't eat cheesecake two or three times a week if I want to look and feel great.

Use your mouth to input great food and to output encouraging words.

God has blessed us with so many wonderful things to eat. I thank Him for not having everything look and taste like Brussels sprouts! All foods are not created equally. In terms of wellness, whole wheat bread is better nutritionally than white bread. Greek yogurt is a better source of vitamins and nutrients than potato chips. As you start adding healthier choices to your meals, you will actually start enjoying them. You'll also love the way you feel. Friends and coworkers will ask you what you're doing and they'll tell you how great you look.

5. Recite positive affirmations twice a day.

The best tool in your wellness arsenal is your mouth.

Yes, what you put into your mouth is important, but what comes out of your mouth is just as important. For several years, I would say to anyone who would listen that I could not lose weight. I declared that I would always be fat. I spoke those words into existence. Now I monitor what comes out of my mouth and even what I allow myself to think.

I enjoy listening to self-help books during my commute. One thing I learned from those books was to prepare and state affirmations out loud at least twice a day. I recite my affirmations twice in the shower each morning and twice before bed at night. I recite two to four different affirmations a day, depending on where I am in terms of goals. By beginning your day with affirmations, you set the tone for how you are going to spend your physical and mental energy. When you recite affirmations before bed, you give your subconscious mind an assignment. You may wake up with an idea that will get you closer to your goals.

6. Log everything you eat and drink.

What you monitor gets done. Trying to save money? Monitor your spending. Trying to get promoted at work? Monitor your production statistics. Want to become a well and fit woman? Monitor what goes into your mouth. I use www.myfitnesspal.com to monitor my eating, drinking, and exercising. I actually enjoy logging what I'm eating and drinking. I give myself a little pat on the back when I drink all seven glasses of water and eat enough fruits and veggies. Many apps are available for you to use. You can also keep a small notepad in your purse. I have a large wall calendar in my bedroom. When I get up in the morning, I record how many hours I slept. These are ways to hold yourself accountable.

7. Exercise at least 150 minutes a week.

If you're not exercising at all, this one is going to seem impossible for you. But it's not. You'll gradually work up to 150 minutes a week. In other words, 150 minutes is exercising five days a week for 30 minutes each time. Or consider exercising for an hour on two days and 30 minutes on a third day. Little steps matter. Park as far away as you can from the door at work or the grocery store. When you're on a call at work or at home, walk around or march in place instead of sitting. Jog in place while you watch TV. Park the car and go inside the bank, the cleaners, or any other business that you patronize. Check out dance and exercise DVDs from the library. You can sample for free! Exercise gives you an instant mood boost. It aids in digestion. Exercise prevents diabetes, stroke, and heart disease.

How do you find time? You may need to cut out some things on a temporary basis. Do you spend three hours at the hair salon every Saturday? Either be the first person in your stylist's chair so that she can get you out on time, or choose a stylist who can get you in and out within two hours. It's a matter of choices. You have to make your wellness a priority.

There you have it, the overview of the Quit Skinny Wellness Plan. This is a sensible, simple plan that will help you make great strides towards your wellness goals. I recommend you tackle the step that is easiest for you. If you already drink five glasses of water a day, start with the water step. I recommend that you add the two easiest steps over a couple of weeks, and then the next two easiest steps and so on. This is a marathon, not a sprint. Take your time. It takes about three weeks of doing something to establish a habit.

QUIT SKINNY NOTES

Use this section to write down ideas, goals, and questions.

_____

_____

_____

_____

Chapter Four

WHY SLEEP MATTERS

"A good laugh and a long sleep are the best cures in the doctor's book."

—IRISH PROVERB

In college, I sometimes got by on two or three hours of sleep. Sometimes I was up studying all night. At other times I was out partying! If I needed a boost, I took some over-the-counter caffeine to stay awake. Once I entered law school, the sleep deprivation continued. Unlike most law students who studied two or three hours a night, I usually studied about 45 minutes each night and hoped that no professor would call on me. I had more responsibilities and fewer resources than most of my classmates.

While I was a prosecutor, preparing for trial was a critical part of my job. When I had a trial, I often went to bed at 10:00 p.m. and arose at 2:00 a.m. on the day of the trial so that I could review the file and prepare my questions a few hours before work. For the next two decades, the amount of sleep I got was an afterthought. I don't remember why I got curious about sleep and its importance, but I'm glad I did.

I bet you're wondering why sleep matters. For years, I aimed for six hours of sleep most nights. During that time, it was difficult for me to reach and maintain my wellness goals. It wasn't unusual for me to feel so tired by midmorning that I felt I "needed" some carbs to get me through the day. A couple of years ago I read the book, *The Sleep Doctor's Diet,* by Michael Breus, Ph.D. He thoroughly explained the importance of sleep. Dr. Breus recommended foods to help induce sleep, such as turkey, and he recommended avoiding caffeine after 2:00 p.m. I tried some of his suggestions for about a month and lost three pounds without doing anything else differently.

As I continued to research the issue of adequate sleep, I learned that sleep deprivation is believed to have contributed to the Exxon Valdez oil spill, the destruction of the space shuttle Challenger, and the nuclear accident at Chernobyl. But closer to home, sleep deprivation is believed to be responsible for over 24,000 accidental deaths a year and over two million disabling injuries a year[6]. Pause for a minute and think about the mothers, children, fathers, and loved ones who died because someone was driving without adequate rest. Chilling, isn't it?

Sleepy drivers are as dangerous as drunk drivers.

Perhaps the biggest eye-opener for me was learning that a lack of sleep increases the risk of diabetes, heart disease, strokes, and obesity. Wait a minute! Getting only six hours of sleep can make me sick? Getting too little sleep can

6 If you want to read more on this topic, check out "Sleep Deprivation and Traffic Accidents," by Mary Desaulniers, at www.healthguidance.org.

cause me to gain weight? Yep. So I bet you're wondering what sleep has to do with disease and weight gain. Let's start with the weight gain.

Through my research, I realized that the reason I "needed" a carb boost by midmorning was because my body was not fully rested with only six hours of sleep. Lots of things go on when we sleep. The muscles and joints rest and the brain recharges itself. A short article on www.mayoclinic.org titled "Is Too Little Sleep a Cause of Weight Gain?" stated that studies suggest that when women sleep fewer than six hours a night, they are likely to gain 11 pounds a year.

In the article, Donald Hensrud, M.D., who is a preventive medicine specialist, said that sleep affects hormones regulating hunger and stimulating appetite (ghrelin and leptin). Dr. Hensrud also noted that a lack of sleep leads to fatigue and less physical exercise. To summarize, when you don't get adequate rest, your hormones misfire, causing you to want more food, and you are too tired to exercise. This is why too little sleep causes weight gain and makes it difficult to lose weight.

Depriving yourself of sleep makes you less effective in every task you undertake.

The next reason to get adequate rest is to prevent disease. An article on the Mayo Clinic's website, titled "What Are the Risks of Sleep Deprivation,"[7] states that a lack of sleep can increase the risk of hyper-

---

7 www.mayoclinic.org

tension or worsen existing high blood pressure. The article also states that a lack of sleep makes a person more likely to get sick when exposed to a virus. Regarding the link between a lack of sleep and diabetes, a recent study[8] found that too little sleep or sleep patterns that keep us up at night and sleeping during the day, may lead to diabetes and obesity because the body's resting metabolic rate decreases. Additionally, too little sleep may cause an increase in glucose concentration and poor insulin secretion.

Sleep is free.
Get yours!

For those of you who are mothers, imagine dealing with a two-year-old that didn't get a nap; the child is a terror. When we don't get enough sleep, we can be cranky too. Several studies link depression and anxiety to a lack of sleep. The lack of sleep contributes to depression and anxiety, and if you're depressed and anxious, it's hard to sleep, so it's a vicious cycle.

In hindsight, when I had the most problems with insomnia, I was definitely anxious. I had significant financial and marital problems. If you are having problems with depression or anxiety that have lasted more than a couple of weeks, it's definitely time to get professional help. In addition to the sleep hygiene tips that I will discuss shortly, I believe that my ability to sleep better is partially due to my taking Zoloft, which is an antidepressant. I don't have a problem with depression, but I do have a

8 The entire article, titled "Less Sleep, Disrupted Internal 24-Hour Clock Means Higher Risk of Diabetes and Obesity," can be read at www.sleepfoundation.org.

tendency to worry and replay my day while I'm supposed to be asleep. The Zoloft helps me calm down and get to sleep. I am not ashamed to be on this medication. If I had diabetes or hypertension, I would treat it, possibly with medication, so why should I be ashamed to treat my anxiety and insomnia?

As I researched the issue of sleep deprivation, I learned quite a bit about sleep hygiene. Sleep hygiene is simply developing habits that promote a good night's rest. If you have trouble getting to sleep or staying asleep, I have

Getting some sunshine during the day will help you sleep better at night.

a few suggestions for you. First, establish a consistent sleep schedule. Try going to sleep and getting up within a two-hour window for each, seven nights a week. For instance, if you go to bed at 10:30 weeknights, make sure you're in bed no later than 12:30 a.m. on weekends. If you normally get up at 5:30 a.m. during the week, make sure you're up by 7:30 a.m. on the weekends. If you decide to take a nap, make sure it is no longer than one hour and that the nap ends at least six hours before your bedtime.

Another way to promote a good night's sleep is to get at least 30 minutes of exercise a day. Although I do still have insomnia one or two nights a month, it is rarely on a night when I exercised during the day. Try to complete your exercise routine at least four hours before bedtime. If you exercise too close to your bedtime, the stimulation may cause trouble sleeping.

What you eat and drink can keep you awake at night. Caffeine can stay in your system for up to 15 hours.

> *If you drink coffee, tea, or sodas, have the last one at least 12 hours before you go to bed.*

If you drink coffee, tea, or sodas, have the last one at least 12 hours before you go to bed. I learned the hard way that decaffeinated coffee is not completely decaffeinated. Chocolate also has caffeine in it, so if you're having trouble sleeping, try limiting chocolate and see if you get better results. Before I learned how long caffeine stayed in my system, I drank caffeinated coffee until 2:00 p.m. a few days a week. After I learned how long it took my body to eliminate the caffeine, I switched to decaffeinated coffee, but I don't drink it after 2:00 p.m. Now I fall asleep faster and feel that my sleep is deeper and more refreshing. As a bonus, I have interesting dreams that I remember the next day.

A few months ago, I met with a health coach to see if she could give me any suggestions for tweaking my wellness program. We discussed what I normally eat and when. The health coach suggested that I have a small protein-based snack about 30–60 minutes before bed. She said the snack would keep my blood sugar steady throughout the night. I took her suggestion. I believe the little snack before bed keeps me from having difficulty sleeping because of hunger. Some suggestions for a small protein-based snack are a tablespoon of peanut butter, a handful of nuts, a slice of cheese, or a slice of turkey. A 5-ounce container of Greek yogurt is a good choice too.

An hour before bed, turn off the TV, cell phone, and computer. The blue light from these devices suppresses the production of melatonin, which the body needs to sleep[9].

Once you've unplugged, have a relaxing bedtime routine. Do things like taking a warm bath or shower, reading something that is enjoyable but not too stimulating, or try engaging in arts and crafts. Your bedroom should also be a relaxing sanctuary. If possible, move the TV out of your bedroom. Paint your walls soft and relaxing colors such as lavender, beige, or baby blue. Avoid bright reds or sunny yellows. Keep the lights dim in your bedroom, 60 watts or less. Keep bills, work projects, and other stress-inducing items out of your bedroom. Try to limit the activities in your bedroom to sleeping and marital relations. Next, turn the temperature in your bedroom down about two degrees below normal 30–60 minutes before bed. You'll sleep better when it's slightly cooler. Don't you love it when it's cold outside and you don't have to get up and go out? If you find yourself waking up hot or sweating, you may need to experiment with pajamas and sheets that will keep you cooler. Instead of covering your hair when you sleep, try a satin pillowcase, and you may stay cooler.

I try to follow all the tips that I've given you, but sometimes I cheat. I often check Facebook and post right before bed. Now it's out there! Once you go to bed, if you haven't

9 For more information on this topic, read "Electronic Insomnia," by Rachel DePompa at http://www.nbc12.com/story/22189097/12-investigates-electronic-insomnia.

fallen asleep in about 15 minutes, try counting backwards from 300, by 3's. If worry is keeping you awake, this counting exercise may distract you enough that you are able to go to sleep. Recite the 23rd Psalm or any Scripture that soothes you. I will also go through an exercise wherein I start with my feet and tell my body to relax and go to sleep. I have a roll-on bottle of lavender that I sometimes rub on my temples and inhale to help me sleep.

If I am still awake an hour after going to bed, I get up. I usually read or do something else enjoyable. A few weeks ago I couldn't sleep, so I arranged some souvenirs on cork boards. Keep in mind, I find organizing things to be relaxing. Next, I have a small snack such as a piece of cheese. I try to stay up until I can barely keep my eyes open, and then I try to go back to sleep. Don't lie in bed wide awake for more than an hour. Get up, have a small snack, and do something enjoyable until you feel sleepy. Don't get up and watch TV or use any kind of a computer, including your smart phone.

If after trying all these tips, you're still having trouble sleeping or if your family members tell you that you snore loudly, talk to your doctor about a sleep study. You'll spend the night at a sleep center, and a machine and a technician will monitor how long you sleep and how you sleep. The sleep study may show that you have an often undiagnosed disease called sleep apnea. With sleep apnea, you actually stop breathing several times a night although you probably don't realize it. People with sleep apnea are often tired during the day and may even fall asleep during the day without intending to.

QUIT SKINNY NOTES

Use this section to write down ideas, goals, and questions.

_____
_____
_____
_____
_____
_____
_____
_____
_____
_____
_____
_____
_____
_____
_____
_____
_____
_____
_____
_____
_____
_____
_____
_____
_____
_____
_____
_____
_____

QUIT SKINNY!

Chapter Five

WHAT YOU SHOULD
EAT AND DRINK

"Let food be thy medicine and medicine be thy food."

—HIPPOCRATES

In this chapter I give you the names and descriptions of the best foods, drinks, and spices available for wellness. Try to integrate one or two of these items into your meals every week, until you reach the point where you're mostly eating from this list. There are probably another three dozen foods that could have made this list, but for the sake of making this wellness program simple and manageable, I chose to limit the list.

If you eat from this list of foods for 20 out of 21 meals a week, you will see a dramatic change in how you look and feel.

I look and feel better now, than I ever have because I started treating my body like the temple that it is.

More than likely, your blood pressure, blood sugar, and cholesterol will improve after a few months of following the overall wellness plan. When your doctor asks you what your secret is, tell her that you Quit Skinny!

1. Kale

Anita Renfroe, a Christian comedian, posted on Facebook that she wanted to hire the marketing firm that promotes kale. Me too! This dark-green leafy vegetable has come from the shadows to the forefront of discussions about the best foods. Kale is an outstanding source of vitamins A and C. Vitamin C helps the body to ward off infection, and vitamin A is good for your skin and eyes. Eating dark-green leafy vegetables keeps food chugging through the digestive system so that you can avoid constipation. Kale is low in calories, approximately 36 in a cup, so you can eat quite a bit of it. I like to steam it with chicken broth, olive oil, garlic, and curry. Partially because of its recent popularity, kale is on most lists of "dirty" fruits and vegetables, meaning that dangerous pesticides are used in growing it. Therefore you should buy only organic kale.

2. Blueberries

As I've started eating more fruits and fewer cookies, cakes, and candy bars, I've noticed that the fruit tastes sweeter.

I began eating blueberries a few years ago when I learned that they were loaded with life-extending antioxidants. In terms of sweets, they are very low in calories, about 80 per cup. Most fruits and veggies are loaded with water, so they keep you full longer. Blueberries are a good source of fiber (to keep it moving) and vitamin C, which helps to maintain a healthy immune system. Blueberries are also on the "dirty" list, so buy organic.

3. Blackberries

Blackberries are one of my favorite fruits. These wellness powerhouses deliver antioxidants, fiber, and vitamin C in respectable amounts. At only 81 calories a cup, they fill you up without excessive calories. They are also on the "dirty" list, so buy organic.

4. Strawberries

Strawberries are an excellent source of fiber and vitamins A and C. Like most fruits, they have a significant amount of water, so you feel satisfied after eating a serving. They are also low in calories. They are on the "dirty" list, so buy only the organic ones.

Go to the grocery store without the children and the husband.

5. Apples

If only one apple a day could keep the doctor away, you wouldn't need to be reading this book, and I wouldn't have needed to see an endocrinologist to prevent my family history of diabetes from catching up to me. Let's travel back to my grandmother's house for a moment. Down the "path" that we used to walk to church, there was a tree that produced small, tart green apples. Usually, a couple dozen apples on the ground waited to be picked up and eaten without ever being washed. Eating those dirty apples didn't kill me. Apples range in size from the small ones at my grandmother's house, to some the size of a grapefruit.

Keep quick and easy meals and snacks handy, such as tuna packs.

They also come in a variety of flavors, from Granny Smith to Red Delicious. An average-size apple is about the size of a woman's fist. It contains about 65 calories and about three grams of fiber. Apples are on the "dirty" list of fruits and veggies, so buy organic.

6. Oranges

Surely you didn't think a Floridian would write a book about wellness and not mention the state fruit! Oranges are juicy and sweet. As a bonus, put the peel in the garbage disposal and grind it up. Your kitchen will smell great. From a nutritional standpoint, oranges have a significant amount of vitamin C, which supports the immune system. Choose an orange over orange juice because the orange has four grams of fiber and only 85 calories; you will feel more satisfied with the orange.

7. Bananas

Bananas are filling, low in calories, and are a good source of potassium, manganese, vitamin B6, and vitamin C. Keep in mind that the browner the banana, the higher the carbohydrate content. I like to have a banana before I exercise in the morning. It's quick, gives me energy, and doesn't have me feeling too full to exercise.

8. Kiwi

I love these fuzzy jewels. Not only are they sweet, but they are nutrition powerhouses. They are fat free and are excellent sources of vitamins E and C. They are also a good source of dietary fiber. I thoroughly wash these before eating because I eat the entire fruit, skin included.

9. Mangoes

Here is another one of my favorites. In terms of health benefits, mangoes are a good source of fiber and vitamin C. It is often included in lists of "super fruits." Antioxidants in mangoes have been shown in research studies to prevent certain types of breast and colon cancers. A cup of mango has about 100 delicious calories and contains over 20 vitamins and minerals.

10. Cabbage

No need to wrinkle up your nose and wonder if I know that eating cabbage makes you gassy. Of course I know; I eat cabbage all the time. My children suffer, but they live. Cabbage is low in calories and high in fiber, vitamin C, and many cancer-preventing antioxidants. Studies have shown that cabbage helps reduce LDL (bad cholesterol).

11. Broccoli

Broccoli is a close relative of cabbage and also produces smelly gas, which is a small price to pay for its nutritional benefits. When you're at a salad bar, add some raw broccoli to your plate. I try to have broccoli or cabbage at least once a week.

Broccoli is low in calories, only 31 per cup, and it is also an excellent source of vitamins K and C. One quick and nutritious way to prepare broccoli is to shake a pound of florets in a plastic bag with two tablespoons of olive oil, a half teaspoon of curry, and a half teaspoon of ground garlic.

Roast for 10 minutes in an oven preheated to 400 degrees. The broccoli will come out crispy and well-seasoned. This is great as a side dish or as a low-calorie, high-fiber snack.

12. Asparagus

Yes, eating asparagus gives your urine a foul odor. There, we've gotten that out of the way. Asparagus is a good source of fiber, vitamins B6 and C, and potassium.

13. Wild salmon

Farmed salmon is cheaper and easier to find than wild salmon. So what's the big deal? The problem with some farmed salmon is that chemicals used in the farming process are then passed on to us when we eat farmed fish.

If you wouldn't serve a food to your best friend's child, why would you put it in your mouth?

These chemicals have been linked to cancer and neurological problems. I can't find fresh wild salmon at my grocery store, so I buy the frozen wild salmon from Wal-Mart, and it's actually pretty good. Salmon is high in protein, and also in omega-3 fatty acids, which are believed to lower elevated triglyceride levels, elevate mood, and prevent dementia.

14. Tuna

When I started my journey to wellness, I often ate diet frozen dinners for lunch. Next, I graduated to deli turkey, ham, and cheese. One day, I noticed the sodium content of my deli delights and realized I had to find something else for lunch. Now I eat tuna about four to six days a week. I have a delicious recipe that is quick and cheap. I like the pure white albacore tuna, mixed with olive oil and pepper mayonnaise, salad pickles, Mrs. Dash, and a little curry. I usually have a scoop on a bed of raw kale or raw spinach. In terms of why tuna made our list, it's low in calories, high in protein, filling, and inexpensive.

15. Lean turkey

I prefer ham to turkey for holiday meals, but you won't find a single slice of juicy ham on this list. Turkey may be a little on the boring side, but the white meat is lean, low in calories, and high in protein. If you have problems relaxing and going to sleep, try having a slice of turkey about 30 minutes before bed. The tryptophan that makes you sleepy after Thanksgiving dinner will help you sleep at night too.

16. Lean chicken

For years, I wondered what the big deal was with "cage-free" and "no hormones" in chicken. Now I'm enlightened. Most chicken sold in stores is produced by giving the chickens growth hormones and antibiotics to keep them from getting sick in their cramped cages. The problem is that the antibiotics and hormones remain in the chicken after it is slaughtered and cooked. Imagine trying to lose weight while taking a pill that is supposed to fatten you up. Sounds ridiculous, doesn't it?

When you go to the grocery store, only go down the aisles that house the items on your list.

When we eat the nonorganic chicken from the grocery store, we're probably eating growth hormones that may be contributing to our weight problem. The problem with the antibiotics is that they cause more and more resistant strains of bacteria to develop, which means these resistant bugs are more difficult to treat. Organic, cage-free chicken is considerably more expensive. Since I started adding organic items to my diet, my grocery bill has gone up about 25%. One way to manage the extra cost of eating healthier organic foods is to reduce visits to restaurants where the food is probably not organic and the nutrition information on the menu is not accurate.

Hopefully, I have you thinking about integrating organic items into your meals. Chicken is tasty, low fat, and versatile. For an easy lunch, bake two large chicken breasts over the weekend, and have half a breast over a salad made with organic kale, spinach, or other greens. You could also make a healthy chicken salad using salad pickles, curry powder, and low-fat mayo.

17. Herring

Of course you've heard the saying that fish is brain food. It is true. This wellness program is about overall wellness, including brain health. Herring is a small fish related to the sardine. It is high in omega-3 fatty acids. It is an excellent source of vitamins B12 and D; however, it's high in cholesterol, so keep that in mind if your cholesterol is high.

18. Halibut

Like most fish, halibut is a good source of protein. It is also an excellent source of vitamins B6 and B12. It is fairly high in calories, over 200 per serving, so if you are limiting your caloric intake, plan accordingly.

19. Pistachios

I like to take these to work for my midmorning snack. I buy them in the shell. Most of the shells are partially open, so I can get my goody without much trouble. But for the shells that are closed, I have found that a stapler makes an excellent office nutcracker. Make sure you buy either the low-sodium or no-sodium variety. Most nuts are high in calories. I usually measure out ¼–½ cup of nuts to take for my snack so that I'm not eating a meal's worth of calories. Pistachios are high in thiamine and vitamin B6. Thiamine is sometimes referred to as vitamin B1. It is water soluble, which means the body doesn't store it for more than a couple of weeks. Thiamine aids in digestion, metabolism, and brain function.

20. Almonds

Yep, these are high in fat and calories too, which is one reason they keep you full. Buy either natural almonds (raw) with no salt added, or dry roasted with either no salt or low sodium. Almonds are a good source of protein, and you can use them as a meat substitute. These are nutrient rich and loaded with potassium.

21. Walnuts

Repeat after me: "Nuts are high in fat and calories." But they are still great sources of good fat, protein, and vitamin B6. I enjoy a tablespoon of walnuts over my oatmeal every morning. A tablespoon has 90 calories, and it gives a nice nutty crunch to every bite of breakfast.

22. Oatmeal

I rediscovered oatmeal a few years ago. My grandmother used to fix it for me with canned milk when I was a little girl—delish! Anyway, oatmeal is a good source of fiber and protein. I usually have quick oatmeal for breakfast during the week and, if I have time, I eat steel-cut oats on the weekend. Regular, quick-cooking oatmeal is naturally sodium free. It is a good source of fiber, phosphorus, and magnesium. Steel-cut oats take about 30 minutes to prepare, but they have a lower glycemic index, so they don't raise your blood sugar as fast. Steel-cut oats are a good source of fiber and iron.

23. Coffee

I like a little coffee in my cream. I love a drink called a breve, which is about half coffee and half cream whipped together—yumminess.

A breve has over 300 calories a cup, so I treat myself to only two or three a year.

On a daily basis, I have one or two cups of decaffeinated coffee with ¼ cup of cream in each one. Studies have shown that coffee is loaded with antioxidants. Researchers have also discovered that coffee reduces the risk of diabetes and Alzheimer's. Experiment with the right combinations of stevia and cream until you can make the perfect cup of coffee that isn't high in calories. For some people, coffee causes headaches; for others, coffee helps relieve headaches. If you have problems with insomnia and/or anxiety, try decaffeinated coffee instead.

24. Tea (green, chamomile, sage)

Some studies indicate that drinking green tea can speed up your metabolism, which would equate to quicker weight loss. Chamomile tea is calming, and helpful for those who tend to lie awake at night fretting about the day's events. Sage tea is good for settling the stomach. These three teas all have antioxidants.

25. Water

Water is a wonder beverage. Try to drink at least seven glasses a day. Drinking seven glasses of water a day will improve the appearance of your skin and lips because you will be hydrated.

Drinking water aids in digestion and elimination of waste. It also helps you to feel full. So how do you get in seven glasses in a day? Start by having a cup of water at your bedside. Sip some before you go to sleep and finish the cup when you awaken. One glass is down, six to go. Drink one glass of water before you exercise, to hydrate yourself, and you should drink a glass while you're exercising to keep yourself cool and hydrated. Get yourself a water

Do something or several things every day that get you closer to your wellness goals.

bottle that holds four glasses of water. Fill it in the morning, keep it on your desk at work, and decide that you're going to finish it. If you do this, you'll consume seven glasses a day. So, you're thinking, "I hate water." I'm not crazy about water either, but I love how my skin and lips look.

Now you're thinking, "I don't have time to be peeing all day and all night." When you start drinking lots of water, you probably will need to go to the bathroom once an hour, but your body will eventually get used to it and you'll be able to hold it for two hours. By the way, it's not a good idea to hold your urine for more than a couple of hours, anyway. Urine is waste that needs to be released. Holding it increases your risk for urinary tract infections. If you've never had one, I'll tell you they are very painful. Regarding getting up to pee in the middle of the night, try to finish the bulk of your water a few hours before bedtime. When I first started drinking seven glasses a day, I always had to get up in the middle of the night. Now I usually make it until about 20–30 minutes before it's time to get up in the morning.

When you urinate during the day, look at it before you flush. If it is light like lemonade or almost clear, you're well hydrated. If it is dark and looks more like apple juice, you need to be drinking more water. The bottom line is that the decision to be well is going to take some sacrifices and some changes. This is a relatively small one.

26. Stevia
Once I turned 40, I found myself gaining about 10 pounds every year. It didn't seem like I was doing anything differently, but I kept gaining weight. I decided to try diet sodas and artificial sweeteners. This seemed to really help. I didn't realize how many calories I was consuming through a straw. Now I realize that the chemicals used in diet sodas and artificial sweeteners are not good for me either. A few years ago I heard about stevia, which is an herb. I heard it

was as sweet as sugar. Well, I tried stevia and didn't like it. I went back to my artificial sweeteners. The more I learned about artificial sweeteners, the more I realized I had to stop consuming them, so I gave stevia another try.

If you keep eating the same things, you won't make measurable changes in your wellness. It takes more than exercise.

Now that I've gotten used to it, I don't mind it. It doesn't taste as sweet as sugar or artificial sweeteners to me, but it's better for me. Stevia is readily available in large bags and individual packets. Check the label before you buy, to insure that no artificial ingredients are added. Most restaurants don't offer stevia on the table, so I keep several individual packets in my purse.

27. Whole wheat breads and pastas

I love soft white bread, but it is stripped of most vitamins and nutrients. It is so loaded with carbs and lacking in fiber that your body digests it very quickly. Consequently, you might as well be eating candy. Whole wheat breads and pastas have more of the naturally occurring vitamins and minerals, and they have fiber, so your body has to spend more time digesting them. You'll feel full longer. Yep, white breads and pastas might taste better to you, but you'll get used to the whole wheat and whole grain varieties. Alexa Foods makes frozen whole wheat rolls that are quite tasty. I also like the frozen Ezekiel and Genesis breads, which are all natural.

28. Brown rice

Similar to whole wheat breads and pastas, brown rice is superior to white rice because it has more nutrients. It also has a little fiber. It's fairly high in carbs and calories, though.

29. Eggs

For a few years, eggs got a bad rap. Now they're back. Eggs are an excellent source of protein and iron. An omelet containing cheese, bell peppers, and some Mrs. Dash for seasoning, is a quick and easy dinner if you haven't planned anything in advance.

30. Greek yogurt

I prefer the texture of Greek yogurt compared to regular yogurt. Greek yogurt is an excellent source of protein, calcium, and vitamin D. It is a good snack because the protein will help you stay full. The good bacteria in yogurt is linked to a strong immune system. Many studies suggest that eating yogurt helps with weight loss, probably because it's low in calories and high in protein. Additionally, yogurt helps prevent yeast infections by balancing the bacteria in the vaginal area. The best way to eat Greek yogurt is to buy the no-fat or low-fat plain in a 16-ounce tub. Add your own fruits, vanilla, and stevia to taste. Greek yogurt is great in smoothies too.

31. Milk and almond milk

I have never been a milk drinker. However, I like to make my oatmeal and my steel-cut oats with milk instead of water. Milk is an excellent source of calcium, protein, and vitamins. Recently I decided to try almond milk. It has only

30 calories per cup and 2.5 grams of fat. It has 45% of the calcium that you need in a day and 25% of the vitamin D. It is grayish in appearance compared to milk, but it tastes great in my oatmeal. It's definitely worth a try if you're counting calories.

32. Lean beef

By lean, I mean only 5% fat as opposed to 10% or more. Beef is a good source of protein and iron.

33. Beans (black, kidney, garbanzo)

Beans are a good source of protein and fiber. However, most are high in calories and carbohydrates, so keep that in mind when adding them to your meals. I met with a dietician once who advised me to think of beans as carbs instead of meats when having them with meals.

34. Lentils

Lentils are similar to beans in terms of appearance and nutritional content. Like beans, they are a bargain. You can usually buy a large bag containing about a dozen servings for less than $3.00. They are somewhat high in calories and carbs, but they are also high in fiber. Since they are so inexpensive, experiment with different types until you find some that you enjoy.

35. Flaxseed

You can easily add ground flaxseed to cereals, beans, and stir-fry dishes. You can barely taste it, and it adds fiber and omega-3 fatty acids. I also add a couple of teaspoons to smoothies. If consumed whole, flaxseed may not be digested, so you would miss out on the health benefits.

36. Avocado

One of my favorite healthy snacks is warm blue corn tortilla chips topped with guacamole, which is made from avocados. You don't even have to make guacamole because it is available in 100-calorie packs. Avocados are an excellent source of good fat, which is heart healthy. They are also a good source of fiber, potassium, and vitamins C, K, and B6.

37. Spinach

This is a dark-green leafy vegetable, so you already know it will help keep you from getting constipated. In addition to cooking it the traditional way, you can use spinach as a salad green, and you can add a couple of leaves to a sandwich. Spinach is a good source of iron (remember the Popeye cartoons?), vitamins A and K, and manganese.

38. Tomatoes

This fruit that we use as a vegetable is a good source of vitamins A and C. It is also a good source of healthy antioxidants. A couple of years ago, I started slipping diced tomatoes into spaghetti sauce. My youngest daughter, who claims to hate tomatoes, continued to gobble down my spaghetti sauce. Tomatoes are tasty in omelets. They are low in calories and carbs.

39. Sweet potatoes

These root veggies are an excellent source of vitamins A, B6, and C. They also have a decent helping of fiber. Compared to other veggies, they are a bit high in carbs, 41 grams per serving, and a bit high in calories, 200 per serving. Try a baked sweet potato with a little butter, cinnamon, and stevia. Recently I tried mascarpone cheese on a baked sweet potato and found it quite tasty.

40. Red peppers

Red peppers are a flavorful addition to omelets, salads, and spaghetti sauce. They are really low in calories, about 20 for a half cup. They are another good source of vitamins A and C. Red peppers are low in carbs and have about three grams of fiber per serving. They are also on the list of "dirty" fruits and veggies, so buy organic.

41. Dark chocolate

Dark chocolate will increase your levels of serotonin, a neurotransmitter that affects mood. I recommend having three one-ounce servings a week. Just imagine candy that has only 150 calories, plus it has a decent amount of iron, copper, and manganese. Dark chocolate is also a good source of healthy antioxidants. It's not as sweet as milk chocolate, so it may take some getting used to. Dove and Godiva are my favorite brands.

"All you need is love. But a little chocolate now and then doesn't hurt."

—CHARLES M. SCHULZ

42. Raspberries

Raspberries tend to be expensive in my grocery store, but they are worth the money. They are an excellent source of fiber and vitamin C, and a good source of cancer-fighting antioxidants.

43. Extra virgin olive oil

By now you realize that all fats are not equal. Olive oil contains good heart-healthy fats. It is also brain healthy. If you choose to eat the white bread served at Italian restaurants, dip it into the olive oil. The olive oil adds calories, but it will slow down the absorption of the carbohydrates from the bread. Olive oil is believed to reduce the risk of cancer and strokes.

Try cooking and seasoning with these spices and herbs:

- **Curry:** If you like Indian or Jamaican food, you are probably accustomed to this spice. Research has shown that curry aids in digestion, is good for the brain, prevents cancer, and helps to lower cholesterol. Curry is a natural blood thinner, so if you are on a prescription blood thinner, you should talk to your medical provider before using curry.

- **Cloves:** Don't limit your use of cloves to holiday baking. Cloves are beneficial in relieving muscle pain and arthritis. Cloves contain significant amounts of antioxidants.

- **Oregano:** This herb that is often used to season Italian food has anti-inflammatory and heart-healthy compounds. It is also known to reduce cholesterol levels.

- **Thyme:** This herb has many antioxidants and it contains manganese.

- **Rosemary**: Fragrant and similar to lavender in appearance, this herb helps improve circulation and concentration.

- **Garlic:** When I was in law school, my great-aunt sent me garlic pills and told me to take them to keep from catching colds. I didn't think my aunt knew what she was talking about, so I used to toss the garlic in the trash. As it turns out, garlic is known to be antibacterial and anti-inflammatory, so I should have listened to my aunt.

- **Cinnamon:** This spice helps keep your blood sugar steady, which helps to prevent diabetes. Cinnamon is also believed to help relieve the pain and stiffness associated with arthritis.

- **Mint:** If you've never kept a plant alive in your life, you can grow a mint plant. Placed in a clay pot and allowed to get a few hours of sun a day, mint will practically take care of itself. You can buy a mint plant from the grocery store and repot it, or use the leaves for a few days and let it die. Try chewing on a few leaves to freshen your breath or suppress your appetite if you're going out to a party or restaurant. Peppermint is believed to combat *H. pylori*, which causes stomach ulcers. However, I've read some articles that caution readers not to eat peppermint if they have ulcers.

- **Saffron:** Some studies suggest that saffron improves mood and brain function.

- **Cilantro** and **coriander:** They both come from the same plant, but the leaves are called cilantro and the dried seeds are known as coriander. This herb deserves your attention. It is known to improve liver function, prevent cancer, and lower cholesterol.

- **Cayenne:** This hot pepper helps you to feel full, and some studies suggest that it can reduce pain. Additionally, it has anti-inflammatory properties.

- **Ginger:** This spice can help settle an upset stomach, relieve the pain of arthritis, and prevent liver damage.

- **Cardamom:** This spice is often used in Indian cuisine. It has anti-inflammatory properties and it aids in digestion.

- **Mustard** and **mustard seeds:** Use yellow or brown mustard as a fat-free substitute for mayonnaise. You can also buy mustard seeds and grind them into recipes. Mustard seeds are a good source of selenium, manganese, and vitamin B1.

So there you have it, the best foods, spices, herbs, and drinks for optimal wellness. There are no miracle drugs here. God blessed us with many foods that taste good and that deliver good doses of vitamins, minerals, and antioxidants. If you eat from this list most of the time, your health will improve and you will make huge steps towards your wellness goals.

As you noticed, many of the foods on this list are fruits and veggies. This isn't an accident. You need to aim to eat five vegetables and two fruits a day. There are several reasons. First, veggies are usually low in calories and high in fiber, so they help you stay full longer without adding excess calories. The fiber in veggies aids in digestion and elimination of waste.

Use time waiting in lines or at appointments to plan meals and write out goals.

Fruits are loaded with water and fiber, and they're sweet. Once you start consciously adding fruits to your diet, they will satisfy your cravings for something sweet.

I recommended buying the organic versions of many of the recommended fruits and veggies. There are a couple of ways to reduce the cost of eating organic. First, go to the farmers market. Ask the local merchants how they keep the pests off their fruits and veggies. They may be growing their produce organically even though they haven't received organic certification. You should also consider growing your own fruits and veggies. It is not that hard. Start with one or two items at a time. Your local cooperative extension service can give you tips on how to start. You don't need a huge plot. There are many veggies and some fruits that can be grown in pots on a patio or balcony.

Check your library or bookstore for books on container gardening. Currently, I have a blackberry bush. The first couple of years, the berries were bitter, but they were decent last year. The bush probably produces about three dozen berries a season. Keep in mind that I don't take good care of it.

Here is what I eat on an average day:

- **Snack before exercise:** Banana
- **Breakfast:** Oatmeal made with almond milk, with an ounce of walnuts, stevia, and cinnamon; decaffeinated coffee with stevia and half and half creamer.
- **Midmorning snack:** Greek yogurt, hot tea with stevia
- **Lunch:** 3 cups of salad greens (baby kale, spinach, or dark lettuce), homemade tuna salad, orange, tea
- **Afternoon snack:** nuts (usually almonds or pistachios)
- **Dinner:** Grilled or baked chicken or fish; broccoli, asparagus, or squash; brown rice or a whole wheat roll with butter
- **Dessert:** Two bite-sized pieces of Dove dark chocolate

On Sundays, I have whatever I want for lunch. I may eat at the Chinese buffet or go out for delightfully decadent

Italian food. On Sunday nights, I usually have a bowl of ice cream with pecans and whipped cream—yumminess!

Eating from this list 20 out of 21 meals a week, coupled with the other tips in this book, has helped me to look and feel great most of the time. For four years, I had to see an endocrinologist twice a year because I was at high risk of diabetes due to my weight, elevated hemoglobin A1c levels, and strong family history of diabetes. In September of 2013, it was rewarding to hear the physician's assistant tell me that my blood pressure, lipid levels, and A1c readings were excellent and that I had lost 27 pounds since my September 2012 visit. She released me from the practice and advised me to have my A1c checked twice a year through my primary care physician.

QUIT SKINNY NOTES

Use this section to write down ideas, goals, and questions.

_____

_____

_____

_____

_____

_____

_____

_____

_____

_____

QUIT SKINNY!

Chapter Six

Set Yourself Up
for Success

*"Success depends upon previous
preparation, and without such
preparation, there is sure to be failure."*

—Confucius

If you were planning to build a new house, you'd make
some plans. You would research neighborhoods and
builders, check out mortgage rates and, of course, save
money and make sure your credit was in order. If you were
going on vacation, you would research the places you
wanted to visit, request time off from work, and make sure
you had clothes and shoes for the vacation venue. You'd
do all these things so that you could enjoy your new home
or have a great time on vacation. Your wellness is much
more important than where you live and where you play.
To win with wellness, you have to plan.

A few years ago, I attended a continuing legal education
seminar with several female attorneys. For lunch, we decided we would go to a restaurant a few blocks away. The two

fit attorneys walked. The rest of us, all out of shape, caught the free shuttle. When it was time to order, the healthy lawyers ordered grilled fish. The rest of us ordered pastas laden with unhealthy sauces and cheeses. When lunch was over, the healthy lawyers walked back to the seminar and the rest of us rode the shuttle. That incident really opened my eyes. If all of your friends are unhealthy, you're probably going to be unhealthy too. I'm not suggesting that you dump your friends who are less than the picture of health.

Let me suggest this, though. If you've decided to change your eating habits and change your life, you may have to stop having meals with your friends who choose not to make wellness a priority. Let's say you go to lunch once or twice a week with coworkers who aren't concerned about wellness. If it's hard for you to say no to unhealthy options when everyone else is saying yes to them, why don't you start bringing your lunch and skipping the meals with your coworkers? To maintain the relationships, consider inviting your coworkers to your home for a weekend lunch or dinner that you prepare based on your wellness goals. This is even tougher if the unhealthy eaters are family members. What if your family meets at a buffet every Sunday? How do you handle this? Before the family meeting, eat a healthy lunch even if it means picking up a prepared salad at the grocery store or a fast-food place. When you arrive at the family meeting, you will be better able to choose a couple of veggies and a grilled meat.

The way to deal with friends and family who don't support what you're doing for yourself is to pray and plan. Ask God to help you get through the meal without derailing your wellness plan. Check the menu and nutrition info in advance online. Look at the calorie and carb count of items such as the rolls, banana pudding, and fried chicken. Decide what you're going to eat before you get there. Once you get to the restaurant, don't even look at the menu. Order the item you decided on in advance. If you're tempted to have something you didn't plan, consider the carb and calorie count. Don't let your friends and relatives talk you into eating something that you'll regret later. I'm not saying you can never ever have your favorites such as mashed potatoes, chocolate cream pie, and garlic toast. You merely have to plan for these indulgences. I like to make Sunday lunch my full-out meal. I usually have whatever I want, including the Chinese buffet. By following the plan for 20 meals a week, I can have what I want for lunch on Sunday and still maintain my wellness plan.

Closely related to choosing the people with whom you eat is setting up your environment for success. Most women are the ones who shop for groceries in their homes. Over the past three and a half years, I have completely revamped what comes into my home. I didn't have a family meeting or make a big announcement. As I learned more about food and nutrition, I let that knowledge guide me at the grocery store. For instance, I really enjoyed fresh-sliced cheeses and meats from the deli. I carefully chose the items that were labeled "low fat." About a year ago, I noticed that many of my favorites were high in sodium. I've never been one to sprinkle salt, and I'm not hypertensive, but I knew that too much sodium would cause me to retain water and put me at a higher risk of developing hypertension in the future. So I initially stopped buying the deli meats. Next, I only bought the cheeses that were labeled "low sodium." Eventually I stopped buying anything from the deli. The deli manager asked me a few weeks ago why she never saw me. I told her that there was too much sodium in most of the things I liked. She said she understood. Changing your environment for success is a gradual process. You didn't form your habits overnight and you won't change them overnight. Be patient with yourself.

At your average fast-food restaurant, the grilled chicken salad has 290 calories and it costs about $6.00. However, a fried chicken tenders "meal" complete with a drink costs about $5.00 and has over 1,000 calories. Specials at restaurants are seldom the grilled, wild-caught salmon. Taking wellness seriously will cost more and require more time. So how do you find money for these extra costs? How do you find time?

In terms of money, take a look at your spending for a few weeks. Examine your online bank statement. Are there charges for a pedicure, the hair salon, cable TV, clothes, shoes, cell phone, land line? I'm not saying to give up any of these things; I'm saying to consider cutting back. For instance, could you cancel the movie channels on cable and check out movies for free from the library? Instead of getting a pedicure every two weeks, could you go once a month? Instead of engaging in "retail therapy" every weekend, could you cut back to once every three weeks?

Regarding the time involved in wellness, you'll need extra time to exercise, shop for healthy foods, and prepare healthy foods. Of course, you'll need to set aside at least seven hours a day for sleep. Where do you find this extra time? About a year ago, I prepared a time map. It's basically a chart that showed me how I spent my time. I had never realized how much time I spent getting ready for work and commuting each way. I was spending at least 12 hours a day to work 8 hours a day. I didn't use this information to condemn myself, but it did open my eyes. So where do you find the extra time?

One thing that I do is to put the more time-consuming tasks off until the weekend. I usually do laundry and run most of my errands on Saturday. If my daughter and I are going to watch a movie at home, we usually watch on a Friday or Saturday night or Sunday afternoon. During the week, I try to exercise for 30 minutes each day, but I aim for 45 minutes to an hour on Saturday. If I'm really doing well in terms of time, on Sunday night I prepare my tuna salad for lunch during the week. Ideally, I prep dinner for the week on Sunday afternoon or night.

I am gradually starting to zig while everyone else zags. Nearly everyone goes to the grocery store on Saturday or Sunday, right? Starting this week, I'm going to start going after work on Monday or Tuesday. The store will be less crowded, and the shelves should be fully stocked. I suspect that this little trick will save me at least 30 minutes. I used to get my massages on Saturday afternoons. My salon is punctual, so I rarely have to wait. However, there is quite a bit of traffic in the shopping center on Saturday afternoons. My next massage is scheduled for a Monday afternoon. I suspect I will save 10–15 minutes by not having to navigate the traffic. I also try to bunch my errands.

If I have three or four things to do, it makes sense to get them done all at once. I save time and gas this way. One trick I learned about a year ago is to map out errands so that I make only right turns. If you think about it, it's much quicker to turn right than left. So this little trick could save 15–30 minutes, depending on traffic.

At this point in my life, I am the "squeeze generation." I take care of my mother, and I have an 18-year-old at home. Although my mother lives in an assisted living facility, I manage her medical, legal, and financial affairs. I plan to visit with her at least once a week and on holidays. My 18-year-old still relies on me for rides, advice, hair styling, and dozens of other things, so I don't have much free time. I've started hiring help. I've had a handyman for years. Bless his heart; he wants to show me how to do things. I have no interest in learning how to install smoke detectors or motion detectors. I know how to punch the numbers on the phone! I hire people to help me with filing, organizing, and cleaning. It makes my life so much easier. There are certain things that only I can do, but many people can handle some of the tasks that don't require my hands-on involvement.

Over the past several years, I've weaned myself off TV. Yes, there are many shows that I enjoy. I like HGTV and NFL football. However, I can't think of a single program that I "must see" during the week. I don't record any shows. My theory is if I don't have time to watch it when it airs, when will I find time to watch it later? TV can be a huge time suck. When I work at home, I find myself turning the TV on while I have lunch. So my lunch hour actually takes an hour. However, when I work in the office, where there is no TV, I consume my lunch in 15 minutes and spend the other 45 minutes walking, playing, or working on some other project. If I salvage 45 minutes from my lunch hour four days a week, I gain three hours a week! I rarely watch TV at night. I have the least expensive satellite TV package available. This saves me money and time.

Some days are very long for me. On those days, I'm honest with myself. I can't do everything every day. If I have to choose between sleep, food, and exercise, I choose adequate sleep first, then eating right, and I don't worry about exercising that particular day. I try not to go more than two days in a row without exercising because it is so easy to get out of the habit.

Another way I save time is by having the same thing for breakfast and lunch most days. I usually eat every four hours to keep my blood sugar from dropping. Here is a sample menu for a day:

- **Breakfast:**
  —Oatmeal made with almond milk, topped with walnuts
  —Coffee with cream
- **Morning snack:** Greek yogurt
- **Lunch:**
  —Curry tuna salad over organic raw spinach or kale
  —Piece of fruit (organic apple, orange, or mango)

- **Afternoon snack:** almonds (one ounce)
- Dinner:
  —Grilled or baked chicken or fish
  —Roasted or steamed veggies
  —Brown rice or a whole wheat roll with butter

I have also started decluttering. I have items in my home belonging to four generations of my family. It's a long story. I also have documents that are 20 years old and that need to be shredded. I'm dealing with one room at a time. As I declutter, I spend less time looking for things. Eventually, there will be less stuff to deal with. One trick I learned from a Facebook friend is to donate or throw away an item every time I bring a new one in. For instance, if I buy a new pair of shoes, I put a pair that I rarely wear into the giveaway box. I am deliberately building a home library, so I give away books only on rare occasions.

Another way I save time is by actually writing out what I'm going to do and how long it will take. I deliberately build margin into the schedule. I work backwards from the time that I need to go to bed. Here is today's schedule:

10:30 p.m. Go to bed
10:00 Prepare for bed
9:30 Free time
8:30–9:30 Put away laundry
7:30–8:30 Manage mother's money
7:00–7:30 Dinner
5:30–7:00 Edit manuscript
4:30–5:30 Free time
4:00–4:30 Free time

2:30–4:00 Edit
1:30–2:30 Pay bills, balance checkbooks
1:00–1:30 Lunch
12:00–1:00 Edit
10:30 a.m.–12 noon Tweeze eyebrows, shower, wash hair, twist and roll hair
10:00–10:30 Start laundry, change sheets
8:30–10:00 Breakfast, Bible study, journal
7:30–8:30 Personal training

The best way to save time is to actually think about it. Think about what needs to be done and what should be done. Sometimes, you have to let the "shoulds" go undone. Also, give yourself credit, not blame. If you are starting a wellness program for the first time or the 50th time, pat yourself on the back! You rock! There is rarely a day when I complete all of my tasks. I try to "put the big rocks in first," as Steven Covey used to say. What this means is that you schedule and handle your priorities first. Ideally, I do my Bible study, and I exercise in the morning for two reasons. First, those activities are priorities, and also because I am a morning person. I have the most energy and determination first thing in the morning. Before I go to bed tonight, I will schedule tomorrow on paper. If I don't schedule important tasks, including relaxing or playing, they don't get done. So take time to think about your priorities. Schedule them and then do them at the designated times.

Quit Skinny Notes

Use this section to write down ideas, goals, and questions.

_____
_____
_____
_____
_____
_____
_____
_____
_____
_____
_____
_____
_____
_____
_____
_____
_____
_____
_____
_____
_____
_____
_____
_____
_____
_____

Chapter Seven

GRATITUDE, AFFIRMATIONS, VISUALIZATION, AND GOALS

Gratitude

"Be thankful for what you have; you'll end up having more. If you concentrate on what you don't have, you will never, ever have enough."

—Oprah Winfrey

When I moved to Florida in May 1987, I planned to stay for a couple of years. I wanted to return to the D.C. area where I had done my under-graduate work. With the demands of work and raising children alone, I didn't have much of a social life in Jacksonville. My church life was either very involved, or I was a pew member. I joined and left several churches for various reasons. For years, I felt that I had many acquaintances in Jacksonville but few friends. I was rarely invited to go anywhere with adults. I didn't feel lonely since I had my children and friends who lived in other cities.

In the summer of 2010, I decided I wanted to move to Atlanta. I applied for a couple of jobs there and had one interview that went very well. Then I decided I wanted to return to the D.C. area, so I started applying for jobs there. Finally, I decided I wanted to move to the Raleigh-Durham area. There was this emptiness that I wanted to fill. I was convinced I needed to move to another city to satisfy my vacant spot.

I don't remember why, but at some point I started keeping a gratitude journal. At least once a week, I sit down and write down 10 things I'm grateful for. My gratitude journal is not a creative masterpiece. It's very simple. A typical entry goes something like this:

I am grateful for:

1. My Lord and Savior, Jesus Christ

2. My children

3. My health

4. My dog

5. My home and car

6. My good government job

7. Hopes, dreams, and plans

8. My law degree

9. Having all my needs met

10. My friends Daryl and Celeste

After keeping this journal for two years, I stopped and looked at my life. I looked at my home, which is adequate and comfortable. I looked at my job, where I am well compensated. I looked at my daughters, who are lovely and healthy. I looked at my loyal dog that won't eat until I get home. I looked at the beautiful Florida weather that I have come to love.

Consider your why. Why do you want to be well? Why do you want to reach your goals?

And then I wondered why I ever wanted to leave. I finally recognized after over 20 years of flirting with the idea of leaving Jacksonville, that Jacksonville is my second home. No, my life is not perfect, but no one has a perfect life. I understood that I could address the deficits in my life without relocating and starting from scratch.

From a spiritual perspective, I realized that my lack of gratitude was sinful.

God has blessed me richly, but I was focused on the few things I didn't have as opposed to the many things I did have. Keeping that gratitude journal completely changed my life and my thinking.

You may be wondering what gratitude has to do with wellness. I believe that wellness is multidimensional. I don't think that you can be physically well if you're worrying about all the things you don't have. Someone will always appear to have more and be more. When I'm tempted to compare myself to someone, I force myself to acknowledge that if I had that person's (home, husband, money, success, etc.), I would also have that person's problems. At this point in time, my problems are manageable. They've been around for a while, and I understand them. The last thing I want is someone else's problems. No thanks!

I think there is value in actually writing a gratitude journal in longhand. I believe there is more of a neurological-physical connection. Keeping a gratitude journal is a mood booster. Writing down only 10 things that I'm grateful for, makes me smile. I've heard people say that it's better to count your blessings than your problems. I agree.

Now it's your turn. Grab a pen and write down 10 things that you are grateful for.

I am grateful for:

1._____
_____

2._____
_____

3._____
_____

4._____
_____

5._____
_____

6._____
_____

7._____
_____

8._____
_____

9._____
_____

10._____
_____

Affirmations and Visualization

"First say to yourself what you would be; and then do what you have to do."

—EPICTETUS

Over 20 years ago, I entered a contest to win a trip to Paris. The drawing was going to be at a club on a Friday night, and the person had to be present to win. I had a continuing legal education class in Orlando, about two hours away, that Saturday morning. I decided I wanted to drive to Orlando Friday night so I would be well rested for class on Saturday morning. I figured I wasn't going to win the trip anyway. When I returned to work on Monday, several people told me that my name was the first one drawn for the trip to Paris, but since I was not there, the trip was awarded to someone else. No!!!!! For the next two decades, I longed to go to Paris, but there was never a time when I had the money and the time at the same time. In January of 2012, I decided I wanted to go to Paris by my 50th birthday, which was a few months away. Although I could earn the leave at

I am reaping the benefits of reciting positive affirmations. I've wanted to write a book for over 20 years. Now I've done it!

work, I had no idea where I would get the $6,000 needed for my youngest daughter and me to take the trip.

I started reciting the following affirmation: "By August 15, 2012, I am visiting Paris and staying for at least seven days." I said the affirmation out loud and silently several times a day. When I said the affirmations, I visualized myself at the airport in Paris. I saw a driver holding a sign with my name on it. I bought a French language course. I bought tour books about Paris. I already had some because I had wanted to go for so long, but I bought updated ones. I did everything I could to prepare, and I left the details to the Lord.

I wanted to go in mid-June, shortly after my daughter was out of school for the summer, so I requested 10 days off. May came and went, and I had no money for Paris. June came, and by the middle of the month I didn't have the money for Paris. I concluded I wouldn't make it to Paris before my 50th birthday. So I paid for a three-night hotel stay in Orlando, with plans to go to Disney World for a short vacation.

The very next day after I paid for the Orlando hotel stay, I received a call that literally put the money for the trip to Paris in my hands! I requested leave for August 8 through August 17. I made my air reservations, and found a lovely flat available for rent in the 18th arrondisement (district). The company that rented the flat recommended an airport transportation service, and I reserved a ride. My oldest daughter volunteered to house- and dog-sit for me. Everything fell right into place.

The day to leave for Paris finally came. We flew from Jacksonville to Atlanta. In Atlanta we boarded an Air France jet. Reality set in when I stepped on the Air France flight. The seats were 10 across. I had never been on such a large plane. The flight was enjoyable, including the food. We arrived in Paris the next morning. Before I could even clear customs my driver called to give me instructions about where to meet him. I had heard that Parisians were rude. However, the customs officer was kind and welcoming. The flight attendants on the Air France flight were patient and nice. Once we retrieved our bags, I turned to my left and headed to the area where I was to meet my driver, and there he was, standing with a piece of paper with my name on it, exactly as I had envisioned. He grabbed our suitcases and showed us to the shiny black Mercedes that would transport us to our flat. During our week in Paris, we saw the Eiffel Tower, the Marais historic district, the Quai Branly Museum, and many other sites. On our last full day, we toured Claude Monet's home and Versailles. After so many years of wishing and hoping, I finally made it to Paris and celebrated my 50th birthday there.

You may be wondering what my 20-year journey to Paris has to do with wellness. I took the time to tell you this story to show you the importance of what comes out of your mouth. When you start speaking positive things to yourself about yourself, there is no room for negative self-talk. For several years I said ugly, unkind things to myself and about myself. I spoke negative words over my life, and I got negative results. After seeing how well my affirmations worked with my desire to go to Paris, I started reciting affirmations about my desire for wellness. Regardless of how busy I am, I take time to recite my affirmations in the shower and right before bed at night. When I recite my affirmation about wearing size 12 jeans, I visualize myself selecting the jeans in my favorite store.

So, how do you craft a wellness affirmation? You start with an initial goal. I was wearing size 18 jeans when I began using affirmations, so my initial affirmation was: "By May 31, 2013, I am wearing a size 16 in Lee jeans." I used Lee jeans because they fit me well. Sizes vary between brands, so I wanted to measure my success with one brand. Once you establish your initial goal, give yourself a reasonable amount of time to reach that goal. If you are just starting this wellness plan and you haven't exercised for years, it may take you two or three months to drop a size, and that is okay because slow progress is better than no progress.

I don't recommend setting goals based on the scale. Let me give you an example. If I weigh myself Sunday morning and then eat at the Chinese buffet Sunday afternoon, I will weigh three pounds more on Monday morning. Now, I did not eat 10,000 calories on Sunday, and even if I didn't exercise, I burned some calories merely by going about my normal routine. So how could I have picked up 3 pounds in 24 hours? Sodium. Chinese food and lots of other restaurant foods are loaded with sodium. So why berate yourself over an ingredient that probably made you retain water? The fix for retaining water is to drink more water to flush the excess sodium from your system. I hope this example helps you understand why you should not use the scale as the only instrument by which you measure progress.

Another way to set a goal and write an affirmation is based on how you want to feel. Walking and climbing stairs was a significant part of my trip to Paris. I found myself out of breath many times. One time when I was huffing and puffing up the steps in the Metro (subway), a Parisian gentleman looked at me and laughed. When I first started this wellness plan, I affirmed that I would be able to climb a flight of steps without getting winded. The affirmation was: "By August 31, 2013, I will be able to climb a flight of stairs without getting winded."

I use my time in the shower to visualize myself achieving my biggest, boldest goals.

Always visualize yourself when the goal is complete. Most Olympic medalists visualize themselves winning. This will work for you too.

Your mind is so powerful. See yourself eating fresh fruits and vegetables. Imagine yourself working up a sweat. Feel yourself enjoying the satisfaction of shopping in any store that you like.

Write down an affirmation. Remember, state a reasonable date and state that you are doing it. It should be stated in the positive. If you want to stop smoking, you would write and recite, "By March 31, 2015, I am tobacco free."

By _____ 20 _____ , I am

_____ ing

_____

_____

_____

_____

_____

_____

_____

Goals

"People with goals succeed because they know where they're going."

—EARL NIGHTINGALE

When you set a goal, it should be S.M.A.R.T.: Specific, Measurable, Attainable, Relevant, and Time-bound. Let's try one. During an outstanding week, I exercise 30–45 minutes for six days. Let's say my goal is "to exercise more." Well, what does "more" mean? Does it mean seven days a week for an hour a day? Does it mean I'll work harder when I exercise? Do you see how vague this goal is? Let's make it a S.M.A.R.T. goal. "By January 1, 2014, I am exercising six days a week for at least 60 minutes a day." Is it specific? Yes, because I am saying exactly what my goal is, exercising six days a week for at least 60 minutes. Is it measurable? Yes, either I am exercising six days a week for an hour or I'm not. Is it attainable? Probably so, if I'm already exercising for six days a week and I want to exercise longer. Is it relevant? Yes, because I am working on wellness and my goal is directly related to wellness. Is it time-bound? Yes, I've given myself a deadline.

Although you probably have dozens of goals, consider focusing on one or two at a time. If possible, try to work on similar goals at the same time. For instance, work on getting seven hours of sleep and drinking seven glasses of water a day because each of these are wellness goals. I heard Dave Ramsey, who writes and speaks on money management, say that discipline is like a muscle. The more you use it, the stronger it gets.

You also want to evaluate your goals from time to time. Are they still in line with your major desires? Are they in line with your faith? By all means, reward yourself as you accomplish your goals.

When I finally completed the first draft of this book, I treated myself to a smart TV. When I hit my next wellness goal, I think I'll upgrade my cell phone. Rewards don't have to be expensive. If you like to shop for housewares, treat yourself to some shopping at Goodwill or the Salvation Army. If you like to read, treat yourself to a day of reading and no other responsibilities. It's a good idea to write out three or four possible rewards for reaching your goals. I have a tendency to plow on ahead towards the next one without stopping to acknowledge the accomplishment. I also like to give myself a little reward for effort. With wellness, sometimes you can do everything well for a few weeks but your size doesn't change. Give yourself a small reward for participation, to keep your spirits up.

If your child earned an A on a test, you'd reward him or her, wouldn't you? Show yourself the same love that you show your family.

Write out your goals in longhand at least once a week. Also, type or print them on colorful paper and place them wherever you spend time. I have my two immediate goals posted in my home office.

Let's try writing out a S.M.A.R.T. (Specific, Measurable, Attainable, Relevant, and Time-bound) goal:

_____

_____

_____

_____

_____

_____

_____

_____

QUIT SKINNY NOTES

Use this section to write down ideas, goals, and questions.

_____
_____
_____
_____
_____
_____
_____
_____
_____
_____
_____
_____
_____
_____
_____
_____
_____
_____
_____
_____
_____
_____
_____
_____
_____
_____

QUIT SKINNY!

Chapter Eight

JOURNALING

"Accept responsibility for your life. Know that it is you who will get you where you want to go, no one else."

—LES BROWN

During my very short career as a teacher, I was repeatedly told, "What gets monitored, gets done." Think about it. The government keeps track of how much money you earn, and you in turn pay your share of income taxes. When you have performance goals at work, you make a concerted effort to meet them. Your wellness plan is the same. If you monitor your program, you're more likely to make progress.

I use quite a few monitoring methods. My favorite is www.myfitnesspal.com. This free website and app keeps track of what you eat, how many calories, vitamins, and nutrients are in your food, what exercises you do, and how

Writing down what you do for yourself every day helps you want to get up and do it again the next day.

many calories you burn. You can also input your weight. You can record your neck, waist, and hip measurements. There are places to record food notes and exercise notes. I recommend using one of the notes sections on the app to record how much you sleep each night. Perhaps the best feature is that this app is social. You can allow your Facebook friends to see when you have lost weight, exercised, or completed your food diary for the day. If you stop using the app for a few weeks, it will still have your information and you can pick up where you left off. I see no negatives with this app. It stores your data, and you can look at what worked when you lost two inches three months earlier. Let's say you've been following the wellness plan and exercising for weeks, but you don't seem to be losing any inches. You can review your eating and exercise patterns and see where you need to make adjustments. You'll also be able to quickly review if you've been getting at least seven hours of sleep each night—if you make the effort to input that data.

I also like placing a large calendar by my bed. It gives me great joy to write on the calendar that I exercised, what I did, and for how many minutes. It is affirming to look at that calendar at the end of a month and see that I've exercised 20 days out of 30. I also like to track how many minutes I exercise a week. I note on the calendar how many hours I sleep each night. Sometimes I'll note on my Day-Timer® when I've exercised because I want this pleasant reminder well documented.

You can also carry a small notebook in your purse, where you keep track of your sleep, eating, water consumption, and exercise.

A recent article on WebMD noted that people who want to lose weight have more success if they write down what they eat. Victor Stevens, Ph.D., who is a senior investigator at the Kaiser Permanente Center for Health Research, was quoted in the article. Dr. Stevens said that the most potent piece of keeping a food diary is accountability. Dr. Stevens noted that the food diary can target areas for improvement. He offered tips for keeping a food diary, including to write as you go as opposed to waiting until the end of the day, focus on portion size, use whatever type of diary works best for you, record what you eat even on days when you don't follow your plan, and cook at home, where you have more control over ingredients.

If you really want to ramp it up, pair up with a friend or relative with similar wellness goals. Get together once a week in person, by phone, or by Skype, and review each other's journals. Knowing that your friend will review your journal should help you to sleep, exercise, and eat in a manner that is consistent with your wellness goals.

QUIT SKINNY NOTES

Use this section to write down ideas, goals, and questions.

_____

_____

_____

_____

QUIT SKINNY!

Chapter Nine

GET OFF YOUR BUM!

"Those who do not find time for exercise will have to find time for illness."

—EARL OF DERBY

Early last year, I found an end table at the Salvation Army that I thought would work nicely in my dining room. The table was only $7.00. I lifted it into the backseat of my car. Although it wasn't heavy, it was somewhat bulky, so my daughter helped me take it into the house. About 12 hours later, I started having low back pain and stiffness. It didn't get better after a couple of days, so I went to the doctor. I was hoping to get a muscle relaxer. The doctor ordered X-rays and tested my range of motion. The X-rays revealed that nothing was out of place. The doctor refused to give me a muscle relaxer and told me to keep moving.

An excellent way to measure your activity is to buy an inexpensive pedometer.

"Motion is lotion," she told me with a smile. I got a Swedish massage to try to ease the stiffness out of my back. I continued to go to work, and tried to do some gentle exercises. After a few days, my back was normal without using a muscle relaxer. Once I tallied the cost of the co-pay for the doctor and the massage, the $7.00 table ended up costing me over $100! The doctor was right that I needed to keep moving even with the back pain.

I went to three out-of-town conferences in the fall of 2013. Two were in Vail, Colorado. As you can imagine, I sat for several hours each day. I normally stand most of the day at work. I was stiff during the first conference and stiff and in mild pain during the second conference. I know that the cold, dry air contributed, but I think the main reason my joints were stiff is because I wasn't moving much. The conference days lasted from 8:00 a.m. until about 9:00 p.m., with only a few short breaks, so I didn't make time to exercise. Consequently, I regressed with my wellness plan. Add to that my eating restaurant meals two or three times a day.

A critical component of this wellness plan is movement. Whether you want to improve your blood pressure and blood sugar or lose weight, you have to move. Let's start with the easy stuff. When you go to the grocery store, park as far away as you safely can. When you need to transact business with your bank or credit union, park the car and go in. Look at this as stealing exercise. Walk down the steps at work instead of taking the elevator. Take a five-minute break from work and walk briskly around the building. In my office, the computer desks move up or down to accommodate those who want to sit and those who want to stand. When I started standing about a year ago, I could only stand for about two hours out of an eight-hour workday. Now I can stand for the entire time. I do sit down for an hour on my lunch break. Make these subtle changes to your routine that won't take much time yet will pay awesome dividends.

Think for a minute about the way God designed us. He designed us to work outside, taking care of our animals and our crops. He didn't make us to sit all day! Over the past 50 years, we've made life physically easier and easier for ourselves. Although it probably seemed like a good idea at the time, *Have we made life too easy for ourselves?* our sedentary lifestyle is actually deadly. According to an article on www.WEBMD.com, research shows that long periods of sitting increase the risk of heart disease, diabetes, cancer, and obesity. Titled, "Do You Have Sitting Disease?" the article states that "sitting disease" is the term for a sedentary lifestyle. The article states that Australian researchers found that each hour spent watching TV is linked to an 18% increase in the risk of dying from cardiovascular disease because of the time sitting.

So how do you go from sitting on your bum all day to moving a lot more? Make slow, gradual changes. Set S.M.A.R.T. goals. Let's say you're not exercising at all. Decide that you're going to park far away from the grocery store, walk into the bank and restaurants, instead of using the drive-through, and march in place 10 minutes a day.

That's a little bit to get you started. Most public libraries have a decent selection of exercise DVDs that you can check out and use for free. I enjoy Jillian Michaels, and Billy Blanks' Tae Bo®. You can also check out Pilates, Zumba, and yoga DVDs. Try doing a DVD for 30 minutes. If you like it, consider buying it. If you don't want to invest in exercise DVDs, there are exercise programs that you can find online too. Or you can buy a pair of walking shoes and start walking for exercise. Gradually increase your movement until you're exercising for 150 minutes a week if you want to maintain your weight, and 180 minutes a week if you want to lose weight.

Never blow off a day, a week, or a season. You can march in place for 10 minutes on the busiest of days. Yes, this little bit matters because you're maintaining consistency.

Like all the other components in this wellness program, adding exercise will require you to change your routine. You may have to reduce the amount you pay for cable TV so you can afford some exercise DVDs. Maybe you could consider eating out once a week instead of twice a week to free up some cash. In terms of time, try skipping TV or social media for a week. You'll be surprised at how much extra time you'll have. If you want to live well for the rest of your life, you'll have to give up some things to make this program a part of your routine. You won't regret it.

Admittedly, I have good and bad weeks. I really enjoy exercising, but my schedule was incredibly busy the last few months of 2013. I provide a significant amount of assistance to my mother and teenaged daughter. Add to that working full-time, writing a book, and getting a business started. When I went to the conferences, I took my workout clothes and shoes. I did work out once or twice for a few minutes in the morning during the first two conferences, but I didn't have a chance to during the third conference. When I have these periods when it seems impossible to exercise, I make sure I get adequate sleep and I am especially diligent with what I eat. I gently remind myself that I have 24 hours and two hands. I give myself credit for what I have accomplished as opposed to assigning blame for what did not get done.

Here is my exercise schedule during a good week:

Monday: 30 minutes of aerobics and weights with a Jillian Michaels DVD
Tuesday: 45 minutes of aerobics only with Jillian Michaels or Billy Blanks
Wednesday: 30 minutes of aerobics and weights with Jillian Michaels
Thursday: 20 minutes of kick-boxing with Jillian Michaels
Friday: 30 minutes of aerobics with weights
Saturday: 45 minutes of aerobics

This is a total of 200 minutes of exercise or 3 hours and 20 minutes. As you can see, it doesn't look so bad divided over six days. As you're getting started, consistency is more important than intensity. You want exercise to become a habit. If you exercise at least four days a week for three weeks, it will become a habit. You'll actually start missing it when you don't do it.

The hardest part is getting your workout clothes and shoes on. You should consider finding an accountability partner. This should be someone who will check in with you a few times a week and ask you if you're exercising and how long you're exercising. You must give this person permission to question you, prod you, and remind you of your promises to yourself. If you don't have a friend or relative who is willing to serve in this role, you should consider hiring someone to help you with this, such as a life coach or a personal trainer. You can also find someone on www. Fiverr.com to prod you via text or email. There are also free and low-cost communities online that can help you find an accountability partner.

On January 1, 2013, I had a consultation with a life coach, Tara. Before we talked, Tara had me complete a questionnaire regarding my goals for the year. When we talked, Tara helped me to see that I had too many big goals to accomplish in one year. Eventually, I decided to pursue four goals during 2013. By culling down my list, I could focus on my big goals as opposed to getting frustrated by accomplishing a little bit on a lot of goals. Once I hired Tara at $100 an hour, I agreed that I would arise at 5:15 a.m. Monday through Friday so that I could exercise before work. To get up at five fifteen, I needed to be in bed with the lights out by ten fifteen the night before. I can't tell you how much easier it was to go to bed on time and get up to exercise, knowing I had to report my successes and failures to someone who was charging me $100 an hour to listen.

This really helped me get going with exercise. I've never disliked exercise; it's always been a time problem for me. Once I got into the habit of exercising most days, I started looking forward to it. I felt better instantly. When I exercised first thing in the morning, I felt I had accomplished something wonderful before 7:00 a.m. By exercising then, I was much less likely to overeat or eat foods that were reserved for my special Sunday meal. Of course, the scale and the tape measure began to move in the correct direction. I started feeling so good about myself. It was great when family and coworkers started noticing that I was getting in shape. If I didn't exercise in the morning, it was hard for me to exercise in the afternoon. I usually get home from work between six and seven. It's really hard to exercise, prepare dinner, prep my lunch and breakfast, attend to household management, and get to bed on time.

Often, I skipped exercise in favor of getting to bed on time. From a time management perspective, I recommend: sleep first, then eating right, and then exercise. Of course you want to get your rest, eat from the list, and exercise most of the time, but if you have to sacrifice one, let it be the exercise. Here's why. If you only get four or five hours of sleep, you'll be hungry and grumpy most of the day. If you load up on carbs because you're tired or you are not eating from the list, you're probably not going to burn them off during exercise. If I exercise for 45 minutes, I'll burn about 300 calories doing low-impact aerobics, but I can wipe that out by eating a large burger and fries or my favorite, a chimichanga.

Add exercise to your schedule for these additional reasons:

1. It will help preserve the function of your joints. The more you move, the more you will be able to exercise.

2. It will help firm your body. If you're a little jiggly here and there, a consistent exercise program will help you firm up.

3. It will help you feel better mentally. When you exercise, your body releases feel-good endorphins which improve your mood.

4. If you're trying to lose weight, exercising will accelerate the process tremendously.

5. Exercise will extend your life span.

6. Exercise improves the appearance of your skin.

7. Exercise will cause you to sweat and get thirsty, so you'll drink more water.

8. Exercise will help to lower cholesterol, blood pressure, and blood sugar.

9. Exercise will help you feel more confident about your body and yourself.

Recently, I asked my Facebook friends why they exercise, and they gave me these reasons:

10. "Because it's awesome for stress management." EJ

11. "I love how I look and feel. I am more energized, and I can wear really cute clothes at 50!" M.LF

12. "I always feel like I have more energy, and I definitely want to feel and look younger at 47. I also want to keep my heart healthy." GLS

13. "I exercise to maintain good health, agility, strong heart health, and to look good." DD

14. "I exercise to stay flexible and to keep my muscles from atrophying." GCM

15. "To go shopping for the cute little jumpsuits, tee-hee!" KH

16. "It relieves stress." WH

17. "I call it my mental health therapy." FBS

18. "God wants me to." BC

19. "My behind!!!!!!" KJ

20. "To lose a few pounds." SLS

21. "I'm going to live to 150!" TG

22. "I enjoy it." MT

So there you have it, all the health reasons as well as an unscientific poll of my Facebook friends. Get going!

QUIT SKINNY NOTES

Use this section to write down ideas, goals, and questions.

_____
_____
_____
_____
_____
_____
_____
_____
_____
_____
_____
_____
_____
_____
_____
_____
_____
_____
_____
_____

Chapter Ten

Where to Get Additional Help

"Needing help doesn't make you weak, in fact quite the opposite. It makes you strong, smart, resourceful, and realistic. Being prideful is a weakness. Asking for help when you know you're in over your head is STRENGTH. Don't ever forget that!"

—Author unknown

Personal Trainers

Personal training is an excellent way to get one-on-one help with developing and sticking to a physical fitness plan. Before you start looking for a trainer, write down what your goals are: for instance, endurance, toning, weight loss. Ask friends and acquaintances if they know anyone. You can also do a Google search of trainers in your area. Once you have a few trainers to call, ask each one who her ideal client is. If the trainer wants to work with experienced runners and you're just starting an exercise program, it may not be a good fit. Ask the trainer what time of day she is available. If she is only available nights and you want to work out in the morning, find someone whose schedule is more in tune with yours. Request references and actually call them. Ask the references about results, scheduling, and prices. Go to a consultation or have the trainer come to you. Do you get good vibes from the trainer? This is someone with whom you will have an intimate relationship, so if you don't like each other, you won't make much progress.

If you think you've found the perfect trainer, go ahead and schedule and pay for your first two sessions. Do not pay for more than two sessions in advance regardless of what wonderful discounts are offered. You'll need at least two sessions to determine if it will be a good long-term fit. If you pay for several sessions in advance, the trainer may give you a hard time about a refund if you no longer want to continue. If the trainer wants you to sign a lengthy contract, request a copy and take a couple of days to review it. Ask questions and maybe have a friend or relative review it too. Remember, the way it starts out is the way it ends up. If you don't like how things start with a trainer, don't enter into a long-term agreement and don't pay for several sessions up front.

Once you've had a few sessions and you are making progress, the trainer should offer you a nice discounted package as an incentive for you to start paying for training a few weeks to a month in advance. Unless you're working with an organization or gym that has been in business for several years and has several trainers available, I don't recommend paying for more than two to four weeks in advance. Anything could happen. The trainer could get sick, leave town, stop training, etc. I had worked with my last trainer for a few months and things were going well. I was paying for about 10–14 sessions in advance. Once I had one or two sessions left, my trainer wanted me to pay for another 10 sessions in advance. I agreed to pay for four sessions in advance because that would work better for my budget. When we had one session left, my trainer accepted a job in another city. She did try hard to schedule the last session, but both of our schedules were busy. She didn't offer a refund, and I chose not to make a stink about it. You want to get in great physical shape, but watch your wallet. I'm not implying that personal trainers are not trustworthy, but I am advising you, based on personal experience, not to pay for more than 10 sessions or a month in advance, especially at the beginning or if you're working with a trainer or gym that does not have a good, long-term reputation.

Physical Therapists

In early 2013, I received a series of three injections in each knee, and I started physical therapy with Danny.

Danny did several range of motion and strength tests during our initial encounter. He told me that my hips were weak, which put extra pressure on my knees. For about six weeks, I had two or three physical therapy training sessions with Danny before work. Danny taught me how to do the home exercises while at work or going about my household duties. After a few weeks, Danny retested me and confirmed what I already knew. My hips were no longer stiff and sore and my knees rarely hurt. I believe the relief I felt was due to a combination of the physical therapy and injections. My only regret is that I suffered for so long.

Slow progress is progress.

There is no point in suffering with pain when there is probably a solution. If your doctor's standard answer to you is "lose weight," you need another doctor. Losing weight may be a part of the solution, but it is probably not the only solution. I have two coworkers, under 50 years old, who have had knee replacement surgery. One is a little chubby, and the other is small to average in size. Obviously, the antidote for their knee pain was not only to lose weight. To find a more compassionate doctor, ask your friends and relatives for referrals. If you don't have any success that way, check with your social media contacts. You should also check out www.healthgrades.com. With this website, you enter your address or ZIP code and the type of physician you need. Depending on your location and the specialty, one or several doctors' professional summaries will appear, which contain the doctor's name, address, years of practice, hospital affiliations, and patient satisfaction ratings. As you are choosing your new physician, pay attention to how long it takes to schedule an appointment for urgent and non-urgent matters. Consider how the staff treats you. Are they friendly and helpful, or do they act as if your presence annoys them? There are thousands of highly qualified physicians with professional and compassionate staff. You deserve one. Don't settle for second-rate medical care.

Wellness Coaches

My doctor's office offered a free consultation with a wellness coach, so I decided to participate. We started the session by discussing my eating and exercise habits. By the time I met with her, I had lost over 20 pounds with the program I'm teaching you. Still, I wanted to see if the wellness coach had any tips for me. She suggested I limit my carbs to 45 grams per meal and 15 grams per snack. She also recommended I have a small protein-based snack 30–60 minutes before bed. She said the snack would keep my blood sugar steady while I slept. The wellness coach had no other suggestions for me. I enjoyed my consultation and was happy to know I was on the right track. I did adopt her suggestion about having a snack before bed, but I haven't been diligent about limiting the carbs as she suggested.

If you are a daughter of the highest King, you deserve the best.

There are wellness coaches who will work with you on a long-term basis to encourage you to choose foods wisely and to maintain an exercise program. A coach is going to be that cheerleader who celebrates your victories and the drill sergeant who refuses to let you stay off track when you slip.

I have not actually chosen a wellness coach to work with on a long-term basis, but I would recommend that you take the following steps to find a coach to assist you. First, ask friends and family for recommendations. When I say friends, I'm definitely including virtual friends. I found my lawn man and my dentist by asking my Facebook friends for recommendations. You may want to check with your health care provider for a referral. Your health insurance or your employer may even pay for a wellness coach, so explore those options. Once you have some names and numbers, have a consultation. A wellness coach is paid for her time and expertise, so you may have to pay for the consultation.

> *"You have brains in your head. You have feet in your shoes. You can steer yourself in any direction you choose."*
>
> —DR. SEUSS

Most wellness coaches charge between $50 and $100 an hour, depending on your location and the coach's experience. Don't assume that a $50-an-hour coach is ineffective or that a $150-an-hour coach will meet your needs. Many wellness coaches work by telephone. I personally like the old-fashioned in-person method. When you have your consultation, determine if the chemistry is good between you and the coach. This is someone who will know how much you eat, exercise, and sleep, so you want to feel comfortable with him or her. Ask for references and actually call and check them. Ask the coach what packages are available. Ask if she offers new client discounts. Once you've checked the references, if you feel good about the coach, sign up for one or two sessions. If things are going well after the first two sessions, consider signing up for additional sessions at a multi-session discount.

Psychotropic Medications and Counseling

One afternoon in 2010 while driving home from work, I felt light-headed, as if I would lose control of the car. I pulled over to the side of the road and sat for a few minutes. I went to my primary care provider and had my blood pressure checked. It was normal. At a follow-up appointment, my primary care provider examined my ears and found a lot of wax. He and his assistant "attacked" me with water and metal digging sticks and removed the excess earwax.

The incident that occurred while I was driving was the first of many panic attacks. They always occurred while I was driving and usually occurred on bridges. Although I had driven over the Hart Bridge for over 20 years, I was afraid to drive over it once I started having panic attacks. I spent more time when traveling to stores and appointments because I had to take longer routes to avoid the bridge. As I mentioned in the section on diet drugs, I had a panic attack on the Matthews Bridge, which led me to admit to myself that I had a mental health problem. After suffering for over a year, I finally got help.

In August 2011, I had my first session with my first therapist, Dr. Wood. She was her own administrative assistant, scheduler, and billing clerk, and she was not good at any of those tasks. Her messy one-room office smelled like a wet animal. She was disorganized and she kept me waiting. I told her about my childhood and how much I loved my late grandmother. The therapist and I also discussed my troubled relationship with my mother. Dr. Wood suggested that I had some features of post-traumatic stress disorder. She advised me to do some research on adult children of alcoholics. She also convinced me to see a psychiatric nurse-practitioner named Clarice Brown, who was under the supervision of Dr. Baker, for medication management. When I had my second session with Dr. Wood, I could tell she had not reviewed her notes from my first session. Her office still smelled strange, and she kept me waiting for over 30 minutes. At the beginning of my session, she reported having some problems with my insurance company. I knew this relationship was not going to work. A few days after the second session, I sent Dr. Wood an email telling her I was breaking up with her. I received no response after several days, so I had to call. She told me she had been busy and had not had a chance to check her email. I thanked her for encouraging me to consider psychotropic meds, and I told her I did not think we would work well together long term.

After breaking up with Dr. Wood, I made an appointment to meet with Clarice Brown for medication management. I didn't think I needed to be on medication, but I was willing to listen. Clarice Brown was a nurse-practitioner and a therapist. Dr. Baker's office was tucked away in an area that was partially commercial and partially residential. The carpets were thin and dirty. The only toilet for patients was always unkempt. The trash can was always overflowing and didn't have the clean and fresh appearance I would expect in a medical office. I even had appointments first thing in the morning and found the bathroom unacceptable. Now, that's nasty.

Although psychotropic meds are known for causing dry mouth, Dr. Baker did not allow any beverages in his waiting room. At my first visit, I signed in at the desk where the glass went all the way up to the ceiling. I guessed Dr. Baker was afraid of his patients. Hundreds of patient charts were stacked about eight feet high in a horizontal filing system. I completed the paperwork in which I answered questions about how I slept, how I felt, and my interactions with others. After a 45-minute wait, a tall, bleached-blonde woman came into the waiting room and called my name.

I followed her to a comfortable, nicely decorated office with an upholstered couch. She reviewed the forms I had completed and asked me a few questions. Within a few minutes, she zeroed in on the issues with my mother. She understood me so well that she had me laughing during an otherwise tense encounter. Clarice told me I needed to take care of the little girl inside me. Then she wanted to discuss medication. I said I was not crazy and did not need medication. She explained that the same chemicals that made me neat, detail-oriented, and loyal caused me to overthink things to the point of anxiety. She also told me the panic attacks were part of a deeper problem, and on a subconscious level I was projecting my problems onto the bridges and panicking. By the end of our 30-minute appointment, Clarice had convinced me to try Zoloft, an antidepressant that would help with the panic attacks and anxiety.

I would take 25 mg for each of the first seven days, and if there were no problems with the low dosage, I would double the dosage on the eighth day.

When I filled the prescription, I had an odd feeling of shame and relief.

Running from a problem may be the easy solution, but it's seldom the right one.

I was ashamed of being on an antidepressant, but relieved that I was finally going to get some help. I had no problems during my first seven days on Zoloft. Once I doubled the dosage to 50 mg, I noticed I was sleeping better. I had struggled with insomnia off and on for a few years. My primary care provider had given me a prescription sleeping aid, but I never tried it because of all the warnings on the package. Next, I noticed that I could slow down and enjoy life a bit. I remember taking a few minutes on a Sunday afternoon to clean my Disney watch that had needed cleaning for quite a while. Getting on the right medication was only the beginning of addressing my mental health issues.

Months earlier I had met Sharon Johnson, a mental health therapist, at a workshop for entrepreneurs who wanted to improve their online presence. We exchanged business cards. I knew I needed Sharon's service, so I saved her business card. Finally, with panic attacks and Zoloft under my belt, I decided to make an appointment to see her. I completed the forms in advance. Sharon reviewed them before my appointment, and was well prepared. She asked me a few questions, and the session was underway.

"Why are you crying?" Sharon asked innocently. *Isn't it obvious?* I thought. *It's 95 degrees outside, and my generous thighs are sticking to your hot, maroon, leather sofa.* Sharon had a receptionist / secretary / billing clerk who was pleasant and efficient. I started seeing Sharon every week. It was a good fit. Between the counseling and the Zoloft, I started feeling so much better. I was still afraid to cross the Matthews and the Hart Bridges, but I had no problems with the Fuller Warren Bridge or the Main Street Bridge. I used to get a little nervous crossing the Acosta Bridge. One day as I approached the Acosta Bridge, I blasted Christian music and sang along. I found it impossible to drive, sing loudly, and get scared at the same time.

Wise women learn from the mistakes of others. Foolish women insist on making their own mistakes.

Sharon was pleased when I told her of my new technique. Eventually, Sharon reduced my sessions to twice a month and then once a month. After about five months, she released me and advised me to come back if necessary. I felt like a new person. My life wasn't perfect, but I didn't worry so much, especially about things that I couldn't change or control.

I easily could have written this book without admitting that I suffered from a panic disorder. However, I want to help

> *It's hard to focus on physical wellness when there are significant unaddressed mental health issues.*

take the stigma out of getting help for mental illness. When I was growing up, my beloved grandmother never left the house. She did not go to the grocery store. She did not go to church. As much as we loved each other, she didn't come to my debutante ball or my high school graduation. By being in therapy and medication management sessions, I realized that my grandmother suffered from anxiety and agoraphobia, which is the fear of leaving the house. Prior to having dementia, my mother would not drive any farther than a five-mile radius away from home. Although she was comfortably retired, she didn't travel, take up a hobby, or do volunteer work. She spent most of her time at home. That's three generations of women with anxiety.

My grandmother and my mother went untreated, and they suffered. I thank God for giving me the courage to face my problem and get help. If you suffer from anxiety, depression, or any other mental disorder, help is available. You may have to try out a couple of counselors before you find a good fit. You may be wondering why I continue to see Clarice in light of how much I dislike the office. In short, Clarice understands me. She is good for me. She is not intimidated by me. So I use another bathroom before I get there. I see Clarice only once every six months because I am stable on my medications. The good news is that I have not had a panic attack in over two years.

Quit Skinny Notes

Use this section to write down ideas, goals, and questions.

_____
_____
_____
_____
_____
_____
_____
_____
_____
_____
_____
_____
_____
_____
_____
_____
_____
_____
_____
_____
_____
_____
_____
_____
_____

Chapter Eleven

How to Maintain Your Wellness Gains

"The road to success is dotted with many tempting parking spaces."

—Will Rogers

I'm a skeptic. I'm the person who pokes holes into everything including this wonderful book. If I were reading instead of writing this book, I would want to know: How do I maintain these gains? What about vacations, holidays, and other special occasions? No worries, we're going to discuss that right now.

The year 2013 was one of the most productive I've ever had. It was also a year fraught with challenges and changes. I am a creature of habit; I need a schedule. I have also been an emotional eater for as long as I can remember. So when I'm taken away from the familiar or when there is an unwelcome schedule change, I have a tendency to comfort myself with food. During happy times, I want to celebrate with food. I enjoy good food and a part of me believes I may never have another chance other than the one before me to enjoy it.

My challenges last year included assuming full responsibility for my elderly mother, who has moderate dementia and stage IV breast cancer. My mother lived with me for about three months before I placed her in an assisted living facility. I had to hire and fire caregiving agencies, interview caregivers, tour assisted living facilities, and perform the dozens of other activities that accompany being a caregiver. Approximately one week after I placed my mother in assisted living, my father died. I traveled to Virginia for his funeral, which required me to miss time from work, stay in a hotel, eat restaurant meals, and miss exercising for a few days.

In addition to the issues with my parents, my adult children need me, which is a blessing, but is time consuming nonetheless. With everything on my plate, I often feel squeezed and spent. Sometimes I feel there is nothing left for me to give to anyone. In the midst of all this tension, it is tempting to skip exercise, neglect my sleep schedule, and resort to eating out most of the time. However, when I'm under considerable stress, that's when I must be even more diligent about my health. Here are some real-life strategies for nurturing yourself and maintaining your wellness gains.

1. Get your sleep.
Speak up and let friends and family know that your rest is not negotiable. As we discussed in the sleep chapter, depriving yourself of sleep puts you at increased risk for diabetes, heart disease, strokes, and accidents. By getting the sleep you need, you'll crave fewer carbs, you will have the energy to exercise, and you'll find it easier to obtain and maintain wellness.

2. Put yourself in second place.

My priorities are my Christian walk, my mental and physical wellness, my family, and my career. In 2013 I missed quite a bit of time from work. I had to borrow leave, coworkers gave me leave, and I had to take a week off without pay. If I had it to do again, I would. My job is my fourth priority, so if my mother or my children need me, the job will wait. On a similar note, I make every effort to put my well-being ahead of my children and my mother. If I neglect my health and get sick, there is no one else to hold it all together. Taking care of myself is one of the most loving and generous things I can do for my family. My advice to you is to make the time to take care of yourself. Your life and the well-being of your family depend on it.

3. Hire some help.

I'm good at doing many things, and I'm a perfectionist. Consequently, I want to believe that no one can do things as well as I can. In the interest of keeping myself sane and healthy, I now have used, from time to time, a considerable amount of help. I had a housekeeper/organizer, lawn man, personal assistant, and an accountant. Trust me; I am not wealthy by American standards, just solidly middle class. I recognize that I can't do it all, so I hire folks to help me. My wellness is important, so I have to farm out some things so I can have the time to take care of myself. There are certain things that only I can do for me. I can't hire someone to sleep or exercise for me, but I can hire someone to organize my garage. I can't pay someone to eat right for me, but I can hire someone to do my grocery shopping. It doesn't make you a snob to have a housekeeper, lawn person, or other help. It makes you human when you admit you can't do it all.

4. Keep a time journal for 10 days.

You can use a virtual tool or a small notebook. You must log how you spend your time for 10 days. I am currently taking a virtual productivity course. In the first lesson, I was challenged to decrease my presence on social media. I went from checking in and posting on Facebook several times a day to only checking in and posting on Sunday. I enjoy Facebook. Some of my favorite "friends" are individuals I've never met face-to-face. However, limiting my time on Facebook allows me to have more time for the important things, like finishing this book!

5. Do a time map.

A time map is a chart on which you lay out your day in two-hour increments. Actually laying out your schedule in this format helps you see why it seems to be hard to get things done. If you work full-time, manage a household, have family living at home, and have any outside activities, you're probably super busy. Perhaps doing the time map will help you realize that you need to get some help or stop doing some things. See Appendix 1 for a sample time map.

6. Vent.

When you're going through challenging times, don't keep it to yourself. If there is not a trusted friend or loved one with whom you can share your problems, enroll in counseling. Most employers will pay for a few sessions of counseling through their employee assistance program. Most insurance policies cover mental health counseling. Take advantage of these services to help you through the rough spots.

7. Retail therapy.

Prior to getting in shape, I hated shopping for clothes. I usually went for the dark, forgiving styles. Now I love selecting pinks and oranges to hug my beautiful body. However, an afternoon in a department store could set me back over $100, so I occasionally go to Goodwill or the Salvation Army for my retail therapy. I buy books, artwork, purses, or dishes to satisfy my desire to shop. My bill is usually about $20. I've helped myself and I've helped a good cause.

8. Buy the jeans!

If your goal is to get into a size 10 in NYDJ, then buy a pair in the style and color you want in the size that is your goal. Hang those jeans on your bedroom or bathroom door so you will see them daily.

9. Help someone.

You don't have to submit to a background check and volunteer to help children. Look around. Could you give some advice to the coworker who is struggling to keep up? You can thank the grocery checkout clerk for being efficient, and you can speak to the manager about what a great job he did. You can offer to pull weeds for your elderly neighbor. The things that you can do to help someone are endless. When you're helping someone else, you will get a respite from your problems, and you may even realize how fortunate you are.

10. When traveling, use these tips to stay on track.

a. Choose a hotel that has a fitness center. Even if you only use the treadmill for 15–20 minutes a day, that is better than no exercise at all. Some hotels will bring weights and a mat to your room so you can work out privately.

b. Choose your flight based on the best times as opposed to price. If you save $100 but end up having to spend all day in airports and on planes, you'll have little time to sleep and exercise, and your food choices will be limited. Don't be penny-wise and pound-foolish. Pun intended.

c. After you go through security, buy a large bottle of water and keep yourself hydrated throughout the day. I also take a few snacks. I usually bring nuts, dark chocolate–covered fruit, and sometimes a granola bar. These snacks are a lifesaver if I have a tight plane change or if I'm running late for a conference.

d. Check the food choices at your restaurants and hotel in advance. Print out the healthy options so you can order without looking at the menu when you're actually at the restaurant and hotel.

e. Consider room service. In November of 2013, I went to a conference in Dallas. The hotel's restaurants were good. At home, I usually have oatmeal for breakfast. However, if I go out for breakfast, I want a big ol' greasy omelet, hash browns, and pancakes or French toast. While in Dallas, I ordered room service every morning. I had fruit, Greek yogurt, coffee, and a bagel with cream cheese. While a bagel wasn't a great choice, it had fewer calories, carbs, and fat than my preferred restaurant breakfast. God is so good. I was not charged for the room service! I think he was patting me on the back for choosing wisely.

f. Special tips for cruising. Yes, you can maintain your wellness plan when you cruise. Just because hot dogs, hamburgers, pizza, and desserts are available 24 hours a day doesn't mean you have to indulge. Start with your sleep schedule. Decide you're going to get at least seven hours of sleep a night. Next, remember that room service is included on most ships. So instead of going to the breakfast buffet, order oatmeal, boiled eggs, whole wheat toast, Greek yogurt, or other healthy options for breakfast. This will save you time and a ton of calories, fat, and carbs. Plan to get at least 30 minutes of vigorous heart-thumping exercise every day. Shopping does not count! If the ship offers exercise classes, register in advance. If no classes are available, hit the treadmill or the stationary bike. If there is a jogging track, use it to walk or jog. For lunch, have whatever you like, including dessert. For dinner, follow your wellness plan. If you need to have room service to avoid temptation, then do it. When you go to your various destinations, sample the local delicacies. Enjoy yourself. Just make sure you get adequate rest, drink plenty of bottled water, exercise, and start the day with a healthy breakfast. Bon voyage!

g. When you return home, ease back into your routine. Reestablish your sleep schedule. Get back on track with your healthy eating, and start exercising again. **DON'T GET ON THE SCALE!** Even if you've made healthy choices at restaurants, those choices probably have more sodium than what you would prepare at home, and the portions are large. So you may have put on a few pounds. Don't discourage yourself by weighing. If you like to check your weight, wait at least a week after you are back on schedule.

11. Don't drop everything.
If you're going through a particularly busy time and you've missed a little sleep or a few workouts, don't toss your eating plan to the side. Maintain where you can until things are back to normal.

12. Broadcast your gains and challenges.
I use Facebook to announce when I've hit a certain goal. I have many Facebook friends who report when they have a bad report from the doctor or a perplexing health condition. Advice, encouragement, and promises to pray come in droves.

13. Teach this program.

Everyone has a friend or coworker who could benefit from a simplified wellness program. You can buy the book for your friend or take some time to tell her how the program has changed your life. You may want to choose a particular piece of the program that has really worked for you. For instance, whenever one of my Facebook friends complains of insomnia, I tell her all the things I've done to conquer mine. Come to my website, www.ConnieClay. com, often for new tips and insights.

14. Remember your "why."

Why did you start exercising? Why did you start getting more rest? You wanted to be healthier, look better, and feel better. When you want to throw in the towel, remember why you started in the first place.

15. Remember that wellness is a marathon and not a sprint.

It's what you do over a period of weeks, months, and years that matters. One bad day will not make you sick but 365 bad days will. Focus on the now. What's the next best step? Do you need to turn off the TV and go to bed? Do you need to rid your pantry of all the junk that tends to derail your progress? Take one step at a time, and then the next step.

16. Eat at home.

If you prepare your food at home, you know what goes into the food and you know exactly what's going into you!

17. Try shirataki noodles, rice, and pasta.

These "miracle noodles" are made from a Japanese yam. They are calorie and carb free. I ordered a box and received two packages of angel hair, rice, and fettuccine for about $25.00 including shipping. Each package is about 8 ounces, but they are packed in water. You rinse the noodles and then fry them with a nonstick coating mix and then use them as you would any noodle or rice. They are fairly bland on their own and will pick up the flavor of whatever you season them with or put them in. I won't be buying these again because I don't think they are worth the money. However, if you're having trouble maintaining a calorie count, these noodles will give you something to chew on that has no calories or carbs. You can buy them on Amazon, and I have seen some at Publix.

18. Celebrate your accomplishments.

I had a fat TV that was about 12 years old. There was nothing wrong with it. However, many shows are broadcast in HD, so sometimes I was only able to see part of the picture. To reward myself for completing the first draft of this book, I bought myself a flat screen smart TV. Celebrations don't have to cost money, though. How about setting aside a Saturday to catch up on your favorite TV shows or to read a book? One thing I did when I first started this journey was to write out what my reward would be for hitting a certain milestone. I've gotten away from that, but I intend to start again. For instance, my reward for exercising five days straight might be to go to a movie. You know what you like and love and what you don't do enough of. Think of ways to celebrate your accomplishments.

19. Reward your efforts.

Let's say you've diligently eaten from the list, exercised, and slept for three weeks, but your clothes feel the same. Treat yourself to a little something to reward your efforts. If you're planning to buy yourself a new suit and shoes when you drop the next dress size, buy yourself a pretty blouse in the interim. Reward yourself with an afternoon in the park, enjoying the fresh air and sunshine. Schedule a massage. You need to keep yourself going.

20. Make a list of 25 fun things to do that don't involve eating.

Some of my favorites are:

    a. Reading
    b. Going to the zoo
    c. Going to a museum
    d. Watching a movie
    e. Calling an old friend
    f. Organizing something
    g. Working in the yard

Decide that you're going to do something from your list once a week. You need something to look forward to.

21. Make a list of your accomplishments.

Your list can include big or small things that are important to you. Force yourself to review the list whenever you feel discouraged. Here are some things on my list:

a. Raised two wonderful daughters as a single mom
b. Took care of my great-aunt in her final illness
c. Graduated from law school
d. Passed the bar
e. Forgave my former husband

22. Make a list of the things that you've always wanted to do, some big and some small.

For the big things, start planning. For the small things, get out your calendar and decide that you're going to do them in a certain month. Some of the things on my list include:

a. Spending a week in Washington, D.C., to see family and friends and sightsee
b. Visiting New York City and seeing *Les Miserables* on Broadway
c. Taking a cooking class
d. Setting aside a Saturday to read all day
e. Becoming fluent in conversational French

23. Participate in a mastermind group.

A mastermind group is two to seven people who work together to benefit each other. You can decide if you want to meet in person or virtually or a combination of the two, but you need to meet at least once every 10 days. Your group could be centered on wellness, career advancement, or spiritual development. Members of the group encourage each other, give suggestions, and hold each other accountable.

23. Observe a Sabbath.

Our Father created the heavens and the earth, and then He rested. He designed us to need rest. One of my Facebook friends posted on a Saturday that she was enjoying her Sabbath. She is a Christian and her husband is a pastor. I imagine Sundays are busy days for them, so apparently their Sabbath is Saturday. Your Sabbath can be any day. If you're very active in church and have other responsibilities that fall on Sunday, you should probably choose a day when you can rest and engage in leisure activities for your Sabbath. Some weekends, I manage to complete all my errands on Saturday. I go to church and come straight home. I have lunch, read the paper, watch TV, and enjoy myself immensely. I'm trying to do that every Sunday.

24. Keep a pair of walking shoes, socks, and hand weights in the car.

Last fall, my daughter had several medical appointments that lasted about an hour each. While she was in her appointments, I put on my sneakers and took a brisk walk for about 30–45 minutes. This helped keep me on track with my wellness plan.

25. Maintain your dental hygiene.

Buy an electric toothbrush. I like the ones that cost about $15.00. They do an excellent job and last about 18 months. Invest in a water flosser. These cost about $50 and are more effective than flossing with string. My hygienist recommended that I alternate between the water flosser and string flossing because the sting floss is more effective at removing some foods. Also, I visit the dentist three times a year; he recommends it for optimum maintenance of my teeth and gums. Maintaining good dental hygiene reduces your risk of heart disease, oral cancer, and a host of other diseases. Additionally, having a fresh mouth and a nice smile makes you feel better about yourself.

26. Plan.

Use some kind of a paper or electronic calendar to plan your workout days. If you write it down in advance, you're more likely to do it. Treat your workout time like an appointment that you cannot miss.

27. Vision board.

For years I cut out pictures from magazines and pasted them onto poster board. These pictures represented things that I wanted to be, see, and do. Now these collages are called vision boards. You can keep it simple and make it 8 x 10 inches, or you can go full out and cover a wall with pictures that represent your goals. What's important is that you look at your vision board or wall a few times a day and take a few moments to see yourself in the picture. I've only been on Pinterest a couple of times, and I've been told you can do something similar on that site.

28. Goals pyramid.

Imagine a pyramid. At the top is your ultimate goal. Let's say your goal is to wear a size 12 in jeans; that would be at the top of the pyramid. At the bottom of the pyramid would be the one thing you must do daily to reach that goal. Maybe that one thing is getting seven hours of sleep a night. On the next rung of the pyramid are the things you need to do most days. On the rung over the daily tasks are the weekly tasks, etc. You work your way on up until you have a visual graph of exactly what it will take to reach your goal. Post your goals pyramid where you will see it several times a day. See Appendix 2 for a completed goals pyramid and a blank one that you can use.

29. Practice delayed gratification.

Let's say you like to buy a new pair of shoes once a month. I don't know you, but I know you don't need a new pair of shoes every month. Start by buying a new pair only every six weeks, and then allow yourself to buy a pair only every other month. Use this method with your eating plan. If you like to have dessert every night, start by having it every other night. Keep delaying the dessert until you're only having it once a week. I'm not referring to a few pieces of dark chocolate or a piece of fruit after dinner. I'm talking about cakes, pies, cookies, and ice cream. These treats are fine once a week, but they are not good options to eat on a daily basis because they have too much fat and too many calories and carbohydrates for our bodies.

30. Fast unnecessary spending.

I am doing this as I write this chapter. My pastor challenged the congregation to fast something for 21 days. At first I thought about fasting eating out, but the Holy Spirit challenged me to go deeper. So I thought about fasting unnecessary spending. The idea scared me a little bit, and that let me know I had the right thing to fast. I am six days in. The other night, my oldest daughter showed me a big, colorful calendar she had bought for my mother. I immediately had calendar envy. When she told me it was on sale for 40% off, I got really excited and tried to convince myself that I needed another calendar. Keep in mind that I have a monthly professional calendar, a lined calendar in my bedroom, a Winnie the Pooh calendar in my bathroom, and a small calendar near each desk in my home office! I love calendars. However, I could not justify buying another one even at a deep discount. My fasting unnecessary spending has made it super easy to maintain my wellness plan these six days.

As I was driving home last night, I was making a mental list of the things I needed to do over the weekend. I thought about going to the grocery store. When I got home, I checked the pantry, the fridge, and the freezer, and realized I could make it until next weekend without buying groceries. I am a little low on veggies, fruit, and yogurt, so I will go to the grocery store and pick up those few items, spend about $20, and leave. Normally, I spend $75.00–$100.00 at the grocery store every weekend, but it simply isn't necessary this weekend. Discipline + momentum = great progress!

31. Give God a "honey do" list.

When I separated from my former husband, I was overwhelmed. I was drowning in debt. I had started a new job. My youngest daughter had just started high school. My mother was not yet diagnosed with dementia, but I knew something was wrong with her. One afternoon I was walking through my neighborhood to exercise and de-stress. A neighbor, whom I'd never met, started chatting with me. She intuitively knew I was worried. She advised me to make a list. On one side, I needed to write down the things I could take care of, and on the other side I needed to write down the things that only God could take care of. I did it, and I stopped worrying about the things on His list. About a year later, I reviewed the list and was amazed and delighted to see that God had done His part. There is no point in worrying about anything when we can take everything to God in prayer.

32. Push a little harder.

Drink eight glasses of water a day instead of seven. Run harder. Lift a little more weight. I work out with exercise DVDs. If I've done the DVD a few times, I know what's next and start the next exercise while the instructor is cueing. I burn a few extra calories that way. You win with the extra effort.

33. Repeat past successes.

Make notes of what works well for you in all areas. I have a lined calendar on my bedroom wall. On it I write down when I've exercised and when I've worked on this book. I enjoy looking back on a month and seeing that I exercised for 20 days and maybe worked on the book for 17 days. Working out in the morning is more effective for me. As much as I like having a gym membership, I'm more consistent when I work out at home. All I need to do is get up, put on my workout clothes, have a snack, and I can get started. When I have a gym membership, I plan to go after work, but sometimes I want to finish a project at work or I want to get home early for some reason. If working out at the gym helps you get better results, then repeat what has worked in the past. This book actually began because I started writing down the things that were working for me.

34. Ask God to add his super to your natural efforts.

When I say my prayers at night and in the morning, I often ask God to add his super to my natural efforts. My natural efforts are limited, but His supernatural power has no limit.

QUIT SKINNY NOTES

Use this section to write down ideas, goals, and questions.

_____
_____
_____
_____
_____
_____
_____
_____
_____
_____
_____
_____
_____
_____
_____
_____
_____
_____
_____
_____
_____
_____
_____
_____
_____

Quit Skinny!

POSTSCRIPT

Thank you for beginning this journey to wellness with me. This is the book I wish I had read 30 years ago. It is my hope that you have learned several simple strategies that will get your focus off the scale and on to health, vitality, and wellness. Diets don't work because no one is going to live in a permanent state of deprivation. What does work is slowly adding good habits and good foods together to create a simple blueprint for success.

This seems like a good place to update you on my progress. In January of 2014, I took a six-hour road trip with my youngest daughter, Jordan. About four hours into the trip, I realized I had forgotten to bring my Zoloft. I thought about contacting a pharmacy in our destination city to see if I could get the two pills I would need to tide me over until I returned home. Instead, I decided to manage without the Zoloft. I asked Jordan to let me know if my mood seemed unbalanced. All weekend she assured me I was fine.

When I returned home, I had a decision to make. Could I manage without Zoloft for the first time in two years? Would I be able to sleep? Could I stay calm in the face of stressful situations? I decided to give it a shot. I knew I shouldn't abruptly stop taking psychotropic meds, but it had already been two nights. I did some research to see what to expect and how to wean myself down. Of course I wasn't really weaning! I am happy to report that I have been off Zoloft for nearly two months. I was fortunate because my discontinuing the medication was uneventful. I'm having insomnia once or twice a month, which is how often I had it when I took Zoloft. I don't feel any more anxious or stressed. I have no regrets about being on the prescribed medication for two years because I was going through a difficult time in my personal and professional life then. Taking Zoloft helped me calm down and enjoy my life without constant worry and sleepless nights. I am able to drive over the bridges without panicking, and I am thrilled about that.

To address my knee pain, I had been on a prescription anti-inflammatory medication for a few years. I was supposed to take the drug twice a day, but it caused intense stomach pain if I took it that often. So I usually took it every other day, and it kept the pain and swelling down in my knees. In January, I learned that raw shea butter was believed to help relieve the pain of arthritis. I started rubbing it on my knees before bed. While my knees are not completely pain free, I no longer use the prescription anti-inflammatory medication. I am scheduled to have my knees injected and will probably continue this practice.

I take vitamins and supplements, but I take no prescription medications, with the exception of the injections. Reaching this milestone at 51 years of age is a direct result of my following the Quit Skinny program. I don't do everything that I should do every day, but I do most of the things most of the time. My eating healthy foods, exercising, drinking plenty of water, and getting adequate rest have helped me to discontinue the use of all prescription drugs. If you take prescription drugs, do not stop taking them cold turkey! If you want to stop taking one or more prescription drugs, discuss it with your medical provider and develop a plan to gradually discontinue use.

I applaud you for taking this step towards wellness. It doesn't matter if it's your first time focusing on your health or your 50th. You've made the effort to nurture and protect the body and brain that the Lord gave you, and that deserves a standing ovation. Please keep me in the loop. Email me at Connie@ConnieClay.com or post on my Facebook page and let me know how you're doing on your wellness journey. I want to hear what's working, what new foods you discover, and I want to know if you get stuck.

One thing that I figured out as I worked on the final draft of this book is that sit-down restaurants are a weakness for me. I have no difficulty ordering something healthy at a fast casual or fast-food restaurant. But unleash me in a sit-down restaurant and I want the gourmet burger, the warm white bread placed before me, and the decadent dessert. Absent situations beyond my control, I will eat at sit-down restaurants only once a month and, when I go, I will enjoy myself. I will relax and savor every delightful bite.

Figuring out your triggers and weaknesses is a big piece of making and maintaining progress. You don't want to take two steps forward and one step back—that's frustrating. So think about where you fall down. What makes you want to overindulge on unhealthy snacks or meals? A big chunk of what you need to succeed is the gray matter between your ears. Think before you go to the grocery store. Think about where you will eat out or if you can avoid eating out, if that is a trigger or weakness for you. I'm taking a virtual productivity class with Darren Hardy, who is the publisher of *SUCCESS* Magazine. He said in one of the segments that discipline happens in the grocery store, not in the kitchen. That statement really made me think. Darren is right. It's much easier to decide not to buy unhealthy items at the grocery store than to resist the temptation of eating them once they are at home.

I am honored to come alongside you on this wellness walk. I am in it for the long term and, of course, I'm in it to win it! Stop by my website for articles and information on wellness. Regardless of whether you get enough sleep or exercise on a particular day, take time to ask the Lord to help you. Ask Him to help you stay focused and to help you meet your goals. Ultimately, your being healthy will give you the energy and motivation to do more of what the Lord asks. May God bless you and keep you and give you the courage to put these seven simple steps into action.

APPENDIX ONE

Quit Skinny Time Map

This is an excellent tool for seeing where all your time goes. Try maintaining the time map for a week, and you'll see in black and white how long it takes to get dressed, go to work, cook dinner, etc. This tool will help you make time for your wellness activities.

Hour	Mon.	Tues.	Wed.	Thur.	Fri.	Sat.	Sun.
5:00 a.m.							
6:00							
7:00							
8:00							
9:00							
10:00							
11:00							
12:00 p.m.							
1:00							

Quit Skinny Time Map (continued)

Hour	Mon.	Tues.	Wed.	Thur.	Fri.	Sat.	Sun.
2:00 p.m.							
3:00							
4:00							
5:00							
6:00							
7:00							
8:00							
9:00							
10:00							
11:00							

Appendix Two

Here is my goals pyramid for wellness. A blank one is on the next page for your use.

Wear
a size 12
in Lee jeans

Eat from the
best foods list
20 meals a week

Exercise for
150 minutes a week

Eat 5 veggies and 2 fruits a day

Drink at least 7 glasses of water a day

Sleep 7-9 hours every night

Recite affirmations twice a day

Here's a blank goals pyramid for you to use. Put your ultimate goal at the top and then start at the bottom of the pyramid and add each step that you need to take.

Acknowledgments

Let me begin by thanking Dana Pittman, J.D. I met Dana at a conference in Vail, Colorado. During the two-and-a-half-hour ride to the airport, Dana and I discussed this book, and I told her that I had been too busy to finish it. For each excuse I offered, Dana had a solution. She literally challenged every reason I had to procrastinate. Next, Dana introduced me to the idea of test readers. Without Dana's advice and prodding, it would have taken several more months to complete this book and I would not have had the beneficial input of test readers.

Next, I am grateful to my daughters, Jordan Ariane Clay and Brittany Aimee Clay. They have endured my many dieting disasters! Each of them also read the manuscript and provided insightful suggestions.

Thank you, Chelsea Reeves! Chelsea pre-read the book, suggested the deletion of some chapters, and a reorganization of the manuscript. Incorporating her suggestions was as grueling as performing surgery on myself, but I am delighted that she cared enough to review my work and make several suggestions for improvement.

Next, I owe a debt of gratitude to Chiquita Robinson, who pre-read the book, commented on the title, and gave outstanding feedback on the manuscript.

I am indebted to Amanda Bailey. I met Amanda after I completed the manuscript, and she volunteered to test-read the book. Amanda has a strong interest in health and wellness, and her comments and suggestions were beneficial.

Last but not least, I thank you, blessed reader. You picked up this book and read past the end, to the acknowledgments. I am grateful for the confidence you've placed in me as an author.

About the Author

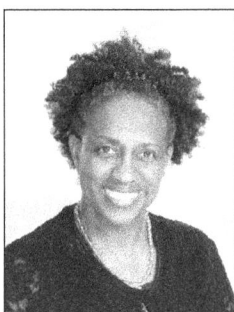

Connie R. Clay's motto is "I've tried it all, but you don't have to." Her goal is to show women the way to wellness, time management, Godly standards in the workplace, and single parenting God's way. Connie believes that mistakes are the fertilizer that God uses to grow poise, confidence, and strength in His daughters.

Connie is the proud mother of two daughters, Jordan and Brittany, and a mutt named Abby. Connie is a writer, speaker, attorney, and serial entrepreneur who lives in Jacksonville, Florida. She was the editor and publisher of *Alberta Katherine Magazine*, a Christian lifestyle magazine that was primarily distributed in Jacksonville. Connie is a graduate of Howard University and the University of Virginia School of Law. She is originally from Virginia Beach, Virginia.

Connie spends her time writing, blogging, speaking, and creating products and services that help women. Her hobbies include reading, traveling, and gardening. To connect with Connie, visit www.ConnieClay.com.

www.ingramcontent.com/pod-product-compliance
Lightning Source LLC
Chambersburg PA
CBHW071131280326
41935CB00010B/1179